Freedom
from
Asthma

Buteyko's Revolutionary
Treatment

ALEXANDER STALMATSKI

with Brigid McConville

with a foreword by
Professor Konstantin Buteyko

KYLE CATHIE LIMITED

Acknowledgements

The author and publishers wish to thank Tess Graham and all the other Buteyko patients who shared their experiences. The 'case history' on Marjorie Curtis on pages 29–31 is adapted from an article that appeared in the *Buteyko Breathers' Bulletin* and is reproduced courtesy of the Buteyko Supporters' Association in Australia.

First published in Great Britain in 1997 by
Kyle Cathie Limited, 122 Arlington Road, London NW1 7HP

Reprinted 1998 (four times)

This revised edition published 1999
Reprinted 1999 (twice)

ISBN 1 85626 335 5

Text design by Roger Walker
Cover design by Prue Bucknall
Illustration courtesy of Armagh Planetarium
Edited by Caroline Taggart
Illustrations by Rodney Paull

Alexander Stalmatski is hereby identified as the author of this work in accordance with Section 77 of the Copyright, Designs and Patents Act 1988.

A Cataloguing in Publication record for this book is available from the British Library.

Typeset by SX Composing DTP, Rayleigh, Essex
Printed and bound in Great Britain by
Cox & Wyman Ltd, Reading, Berkshire

FREEDOM FROM ASTHMA

Alexander (Sasha) Stalmatski was trained by Professor Konstantin Buteyko and worked with him in Russia for 14 years. He brought the Buteyko Method to the West in 1990, working in Australia for six years. During this time he treated about 6,000 asthmatics and trained 45 Buteyko practitioners. Now based at the Hale Clinic in London, he represents Professor Buteyko and his method outside Russia.

Contents

Important Note

The information given in this book is intended for general guidance and is not a substitute for individual diagnosis or treatment by a qualified practitioner or medical doctor. Always consult a medical doctor and qualified practitioner before embarking on any treatment. The reader is strongly advised not to attempt self-treatment for any serious or long-term complaint without consulting a medical doctor or qualified practitioner. Neither the author, the publishers nor the Hale Clinic can be held responsible for any adverse reaction to the recommendations contained in this book, which are followed entirely at the reader's own risk.

Information about Buteyko courses and Buteyko practitioners in the UK, Europe, Australia and New Zealand can be obtained from the Hale Clinic, 7 Park Crescent, London W1N 3HE, tel. 0990 168146 or the author on tel. 01523 192111. Australian readers can also contact tel. (02) 935 72236.

All bona fide Buteyko practitioners offer a money-back guarantee of substantial improvement for every patient they have agreed to treat, no matter what the complaint.

by Professor Konstantin Buteyko

On 7 October 1952 I happened to be the first scientist in the world to discover the major cause of a number of diseases of the respiratory, hormonal, cardiovascular and nervous systems which were incurable by modern medicine. Forty-five years of scientific research and practical work on my method (known in the West as the Buteyko Method) allow me to claim that this drug-free method is perfectly safe and immeasurably more effective than traditional drug treatment of many chronic disorders – especially asthma. Scientific trials of my 'method' in the treatment of asthma (in Russia in 1968 and 1981, and in Australia in 1994–95) showed results unseen in the whole of medical history and proved the accuracy of the observations I first made forty-five years ago.

While my method is very popular in Russia, Australia and New Zealand, in Europe it is relatively new and largely unknown – yet. Therefore I am glad that this book – written by one of my best pupils and practitioners, Sasha Stalmatski – will tell readers of my discovery. I hope that in time a Buteyko practitioner will be found on every corner and my treatment will be available to all.

I bless this book and hope that it will change the lives of many sufferers.

Professor Konstantin Buteyko
Moscow
July 1997

CHAPTER ONE

Introducing Buteyko:
The Man and the Method

This is the story of a sensational and revolutionary discovery, a discovery that could enable millions of people the world over to protect themselves against one of the most insidious epidemics of our time. Not AIDS, but asthma. While doctors and patients are fighting a losing battle against this rampant disease, desperately treating the symptoms because they do not know the cause, the observations of a Russian medical scientist, Dr Konstantin Buteyko, enable us not only to understand asthma but to prevent it.

What has come to be known as the Buteyko method is simply a course of exercises to retrain our breathing patterns, and is an effective and drug-free treatment for asthma – and some 150 other disorders.

Asthma is a breathing disorder

In our culture there is a widespread assumption that deep breathing is good for us because it increases our oxygen intake. In fact the reverse is true: the **more** you breathe, the **less** oxygen actually gets to the cells of your body.

This is because the air around you contains a much

smaller proportion of carbon dioxide than your own body. Carbon dioxide is essential for your body's uptake of oxygen. Breathing too much, or **overbreathing**, results in a deficit of carbon dioxide which reduces the level of oxygen in your blood and tissues – affecting the function of every system in your body. Retrain your breathing and you will cure your asthma. It is as simple as that.

'Mad' enough to be brilliant?

Professor Buteyko's theory about overbreathing overturns many of the assumptions of modern medicine (and modern drug therapy). Some people reading this book may shake their heads and say, 'That Professor Buteyko must be mad! Everyone knows that it is not like that!'

However, the history of medicine shows that new discoveries have often been condemned as 'mad'. Take the Hungarian obstetrician and surgeon Ignaz Semmelweis, who in 1846 discovered the causes of sepsis – the invasion of the body by 'rotting' bacteria. In the 1890s, an average of 13 women a day died in England and Wales of an infection known as 'childbed fever' after giving birth. Today, largely thanks to our knowledge of antiseptics, the figure has plummeted to one maternal death a week – despite the fact that twice as many women are giving birth.

Semmelweis put forward a theory that doctors should wash their hands before delivering babies and before performing surgery. His 'mad' idea earned him ridicule, rejection and, ultimately, confinement in a lunatic asylum, where he died. Sadly, it was to be another half century before his emphasis on handwashing was widely adopted by doctors.

It was Niels Bohr, the founder of nuclear physics, who said that for a discovery to be brilliant it had to be crazy. So when people say Professor Buteyko 'must be mad', it is worth considering whether his ideas are 'mad' enough to be truly brilliant. Certainly his fundamental and far-reaching theory has been met with scepticism (at the very least) by many modern doctors and asthma specialists.

Professor Who?

'Who is this Professor Buteyko?' people often ask me. 'I have never heard of him. And why – if it so good – is his method not more widely recognised?'

I reply that Professor Buteyko is a Russian, and as well-known in Russia as the Queen Mother is in Britain. But just as very few people in Russia have ever heard of the Queen Mother, very few people in Britain – or anywhere else in the western world – have yet heard of Professor Buteyko.

There are complex historical and political reasons too for Professor Buteyko being relatively 'unknown' in the western world. For many years his mail was intercepted, his telephone was bugged and his work was classified as a 'state secret'. He was not free to travel or to talk about his ideas in the west. Buteyko is not as famous as Sakharov or Solzhenitsyn, but he had the weight of the Russian medical establishment against him. He suffered ridicule in his own country for his ideas and at one point the state tried to incarcerate him in a mental hospital. Fortunately he was saved by a senior member of the Communist Party whom he had treated successfully.

Nonetheless, Professor Buteyko made many discoveries

which turned the whole range of medical treatments on its head. It was some 45 years ago that, as a young intern working in a hospital for terminally ill patients, he observed that an increase in breathing was an indicator of approaching death. He realised that he could predict the time of death by monitoring patients' breathing patterns, and that deepening breathing was linked to a wide range of diseases and chronic conditions.

Over the years, Buteyko studied hundreds of patients and developed the theory that much ill health is the result of the body's defence mechanisms trying to compensate for lack of carbon dioxide. Deep breathing he argued, was not just a symptom, but a cause of illnesses ranging from cardiac problems to breathing disorders.

He not only discovered that **overbreathing**, or hyper-ventilation, is the cause of asthma; he also developed a method of measuring breathing and the connections between carbon dioxide, hyperventilation and bronchospasm – the involuntary contraction of the bronchial (lung) tubes which is part of the cause of an asthma attack.

He explained many phenomena which medicine had been unable to understand for hundreds of years – such as exercise-induced asthma, nocturnal asthma, emotional asthma and the links between asthma, stress and infections. Professor Buteyko has also explained why the modern medical concept of asthma treatment is wrong and has pointed out the detrimental effects of asthma drugs past and present. He has explained why steroids (in the correct quantities) can help asthmatics – and (in overdose) can also destroy them.

In addition, Professor Buteyko has shown the connections between overbreathing and a whole host of other complaints including allergy, anxiety, panic attacks, nasal problems, eczema, headaches, emphysema, bronchitis and hay fever. He has explained why people die from asthma – and how this can be prevented.

His method of retraining breathing involves a series of exercises designed to restore normal breathing patterns by retraining the body's respiratory centre in the brain. This – in a nutshell – is the Buteyko method, which can provide an effective self-management treatment not only for asthma but for allergies, insomnia, bronchitis, anxiety, migraines, high blood pressure, haemorrhoids – to name a few. Even the world-wide problem of blocked noses and snoring can benefit from the Buteyko method!

Buteyko on trial

Another major reason why the Buteyko method is not pro-claimed as a success by the asthma experts is that it is a **drug-free** treatment, and as such it poses a serious threat to the profits of drug companies and pharmacists around the world, as well as to the reputations of doctors, hospitals and academics everywhere.

An important aspect to the comparatively low profile of the Buteyko method in the western world has been the extreme reluctance of asthma 'specialists' to consider the evidence of its effectiveness. The initial reaction of the Australian Asthma Foundation was to issue a special warning that the Buteyko method was dangerous. Then it admitted that for every successful Buteyko treatment of asthma, there is one case which is not successful – suggest-ing that Buteyko has a 50 per cent success rate! Not bad for something that has been written off as dangerous!

In 1993 the Australian Asthma Foundation agreed to observe a Buteyko workshop in Adelaide, on the condition that the results of their observations remain confidential. In this workshop of 36 participants, including people suffering from severe asthma and emphysema, **everybody** derived some benefit from the Buteyko method (including two observers, one of whom got rid of a blocked nose problem while the other learned how to overcome and then prevent her own asthma attacks).

The Australian Asthma Campaign observed another Buteyko workshop in Melbourne, during May 1994. Data from this workshop was analysed by Professor Charles Mitchell, an internationally respected asthma specialist, who in October 1994 advised that as a result of the Buteyko method, '75 per cent of participants reported that asthma symptoms occurred less frequently, and 90 per cent had been able to reduce their medication'. Professor Mitchell also sent three of his severely asthmatic patients to learn the Buteyko method, and reported that they derived great benefit from this treatment within one week.

In 1994 an eight-month scientific trial was at last set up by the Australian Asthma Foundation after intense pressure from the public and the media to investigate the Buteyko method. It followed a period of many years during which asthma specialists had tried to ignore or discredit the Buteyko method.

This trial was conducted at the Mater Hospital, Brisbane, in 1994–5 (see Appendix page 177). The result was a 90 per cent reduction in the use of bronchodilators and a 49 per cent reduction in the use of steroids by participants in the trial. The leading medical magazine

Australian Doctor published two articles on the trial entitled 'Doctors Gasp at Buteyko Success' and 'Buteyko Lowers Need for Drugs'.

Disappointingly, these entirely positive results were not communicated to the public by the Australian Asthma Foundation. It seemed that some doctors were willing to prescribe asthma drugs without understanding fully how they worked, yet they were not willing to try the Buteyko method – because they didn't understand fully how it worked.

Fortunately, many Australians discovered for themselves that the Buteyko method is effective and the network of Buteyko teachers and supporters grew fast – but the same story of suspicion and reluctance to accept the success of Buteyko treatments was repeated here in Britain.

In Australia and New Zealand it is the media (as well as people successfully treated by the Buteyko method) who have spread the news that now there is a treatment which can stop asthma, once and for all. And again, this pattern is being repeated in Britain, where reputable journals have called for asthma specialists not to dismiss a potential cure for asthma out of hand.

In December 1998 the *Medical Journal of Australia* finally published a report on the trial (see Bowler et al in References, page 183). The editorial comment on the report was cautious, calling for more rigorous, high-quality clinical trials of 'unproven' therapies. It observed that Buteyko had provided 'no benefit...on objective measures of asthma', but remarked on the 'significant reduction in the self-reported use of short-acting bronchodilators and trends for reduction in the self-reported use of inhaled steroids and for improved quality of life.' It went on to say:

Overall, the study showed no improvement in the clinical severity of asthma in the BBT [Buteyko Breathing Technique] group, but there was a significant reduction in the use of beta$_2$-agonists. These data indicate that some patients can cope with less medication and suffer no loss of control of their asthma. If this is the case generally, then many patients are taking unnecessary medication, leading to increases in adverse effects and expenses for these drugs. Medical practitioners should review regularly the asthma therapy of their patients and consider dosage reductions.

Let us hope that this is the start of official recognition for the Buteyko method.

Is the Buteyko method a cure?

What I can say very clearly is that the Buteyko method is the **best known route to a cure**. After two or three days of Buteyko treatment you will be able to reduce your medication by 40 to 50 per cent – because of the improvement in your condition. After a few more days, you should be able to reduce your medication by 80 to 100 per cent. After a few weeks (for children), or a few months (for severe, chronic asthmatics) you will be able to live without medications **and** without asthma attacks.

This is the best method of asthma management ever discovered. And what a contrast to modern medicine which leads asthmatics to a dead end of long-term treatment without solving the problem.

CHAPTER TWO

Success with Buteyko

So what is the Buteyko method in practice, and what happens when you or your child joins in a Buteyko workshop? The science of Buteyko is sophisticated, but as the success of the method with small children shows, you don't have to understand the technical details fully to experience a dramatic and rapid improvement in your health.

So let's hear from some individuals who have tried the Buteyko method, discovered that it can stop asthma in its tracks and that their need for asthma medications has almost (or entirely) disappeared.

Tess Graham, a physiotherapist who lives in Canberra, has two children with asthma. But after attending a Buteyko workshop, their symptoms disappeared. Tess has since trained as a Buteyko practitioner and teacher, and she now teaches the Buteyko method full-time:

I first read about the Buteyko method in a health magazine. It was all so logical that it immediately made sense to me. As a physio I had worked with people with asthma for many years, believing they could never get completely better. **Physiotherapy traditionally teaches deep breathing** and coughing exercises, but I could see that these made asthma worse.

I was very shocked when I found that two out of three of my own children had asthma, even though this problem doesn't run in my family. My daughter Jessie was so ill that she had asthma symptoms daily and was on inhaled steroids and a puffer (bronchodilator drug). She had been on a nebuliser one week in every three. [We will hear more about these treatments in Chapter Seven.] My son's asthma was worse in the springtime, so at times I had two of them suffering from coughing, wheezing and asthma attacks – which meant not much sleep for me either!

But it was Jessie who I felt was really on the edge, and for years I lived in fear for her life. Her asthma could come on quickly and I wouldn't be more than five minutes away from her at any time. But that was before we discovered Buteyko. Our first experience was with individual sessions, and then later we attended a group workshop.

Day one: a radical rethink

Jessie was seven years old when I took her to the Buteyko workshop. There were about ten other wheezy children and a lot of nervous parents, many of whom had been told by their doctors that the Buteyko method wouldn't work. Some were very sceptical and were holding onto their receipts very tightly!

It began with the practitioner, Sasha Stalmatski, introducing the Buteyko method and honouring Professor Buteyko for his achievements. We went on to discuss the basics of breathing and what he called the 'propaganda of deep breathing'. He said, 'Hands up those of you who think deep breathing is good for you', and about 90 per cent of the people put their hands up.

He went on to explain how deep breathing causes us problems. We discussed how even blowing up balloons can make you feel dizzy, and how blowing very hard into a peak flow meter can make you cough and make your chest tighten up. We soon got the idea that deep breathing is the root cause of asthma.

From that point the children were put into groups to practise breathing gently and quietly through their noses – having first been taught a breath holding exercise which unblocks their noses. Jessie used to be a chronic mouth breather, and there were other kids in the group with gold-fish-type mouth postures from years of being open-mouthed.

Much of that first session was about reminding the children to shut their mouths. If their noses got blocked they repeated the unblocking exercise. If their noses weren't blocked, they were opening their mouths from habit.

At the end of that first session, the change was remarkable. The noisy breathing and coughing, the snorting and blowing had stopped. The room was quiet, the mouths were shut. You could have heard a pin drop. I saw this sea of faces, mouths closed.

I remember leaving that first session with a sense of unbelievable relief. For years I had felt the fear rise when I heard Jessie start to cough, and now I knew we could get out of this mess. At last I understood what caused her asthma and I was instantly less fearful for her.

That first night I followed Sasha's instructions to get her to sleep with her mouth shut. We had some exercises to do before bed to make sure that her nose was open and I put the head of my bed next to hers in an L shape so that I could close her mouth through the night, holding her lips together if necessary and moving her chin.

I kept her lying on her side and made sure she kept her mouth shut. I heard her change from noisy breathing to very quiet nasal breathing. This can be a little bit frightening for mothers at first, because we are so used to listening out for the heavy breathing which reassures us that they are still alive – but I soon learned to love the quietness!

Day two: delight and excitement...

Day two is pretty exciting because parents and children come back to the class keen to share their experience. They say things like, 'He used to grind his teeth and wake up frequently – but last night he didn't'. Or, 'My kid had the best sleep for years', or 'My kid didn't wake up last night, whereas he usually wakes up about four times'. Parents often say their children used to be very restless at night, with a sweaty head and lots of kicking and coughing, but after doing Buteyko they sleep so peacefully that they can share a bed with them – without getting kicked all night.

Some parents say their child's bed used to be like a battleground in the morning, or that they had nightmares, or that they used to wet the bed. Once they learn to sleep with their mouths closed and breathing gently, **all that changes**. They say, 'He played soccer for the first time without his puffer' or 'Mary woke up today and didn't need to blow her nose – whereas she usually needs about ten tissues'.

It often happens that – even on day two – parents say,

'My child didn't need to use his puffer for the first time in years'. In one recent workshop there was an eleven-year-old boy who had been on a nebuliser two or three times a day since the age of three. Mother and child told me that that day – which was only day two of the workshop – was the first day in eight years that he hadn't needed that nebuliser. They both had the biggest smiles on their faces...

On day two it can still feel quite awkward and the practitioner has to remind the kids a lot to shut their mouths. But already they have made progress because on day one some would have felt suffocated by having to close their mouths. On day two it may still be uncomfortable (in which case they do the nose unblocking exercises), but often they are opening their mouths because of long habit. It can be difficult but I've never seen a child get upset during a workshop. I have seen parents in tears however – but those are tears of relief.

Days three and four: work hard but play too!

These two days follow much the pattern. We increase the intensity of the exercises, depending on how well the patients are doing and how much they can handle. It is a matter of fine tuning, which is why you should only do Buteyko with the help of a qualified practitioner.

The group have been doing 'homework' and keeping scores on their exercises. Children come up and say, 'Look! This is my best score so far!' They think it is great fun because kids tend to be a bit competitive, but I stress that we are all different and they are only competing against themselves.

One of the most exciting things to emerge at about this

time is the amazing changes in their pulse rates. Some children come in at the start of the week with pulse rates from 80 beats a minute up to around 130. Adults are often between 80 and 100 beats a minute – which indicates that they are pretty unwell. And we don't take the pulses until they have been sitting in the workshop for about half an hour, so it isn't because they have rushed to get there.

But by the end of the first session, after half an hour of Buteyko exercises, most pulses have dropped by at least 10 beats – and sometimes 20 – per minute. By the end of the week they are down to a good healthy resting pulse of between 60 and 80 beats per minute. That happens to everybody who does Buteyko because if you normalise your breathing the whole system becomes more efficient and less stressed – which means that the heart can slow down. This is one of the strongest indicators of the success of Buteyko and no one can say it is an imagined, placebo effect.

Another wonderful 'side effect' is that people who were overweight have often lost weight, because Buteyko helps your whole system to regulate itself, making changes in your metabolism and appetite. Alternatively, people who need to put on weight find they have gained a few pounds without trying to do so.

On day three we also learn some variations on the basic Buteyko 'breath-holding' exercises, and we apply these exercises to practical situations such as being at school (for children) or at work (for adults). Eating, sleeping, being in a smoky room, walking out of a building into cold weather: all these are part of ordinary life and we discuss what you need to do to keep your breathing under control.

We do role playing to help children understand what they can do if they are on the soccer field when they need to do their exercises, or in a classroom with a cranky teacher who won't let them do Buteyko. Sometimes the children jog around the room so that we can teach them how to breathe correctly when they are playing sports.

For adults, it may be a matter of pretending they are walking upstairs on the way to work: what happens when you get to the third stair and feel you really have to open your mouth? Even talking a lot – on the phone, or giving a presentation – can increase breathing, so we teach various techniques on how to control breathing. One of the solutions includes taking your puffer around with you.

The group dynamic is very important in the workshop because people encourage each other. Sometimes people have slow days or days when they feel tired, but others will say, 'I had a slow day yesterday, but today I feel wonderful'. Or, 'I felt like that, but then I had a breakthrough...' In my group, people come back from earlier workshops to support us – and to show off a little!

Day five: where do we go from here?

On day five parents are commenting on the changes in colour amongst the children: the red ones are paler while the pale ones have got pinker. They say, 'He looks a different person'. The feeling amongst the parents is that, having seen the change in their own child, they want everyone to know about Buteyko. They have this simple knowledge and they feel almost like evangelists: they want to spread the word. In our area (Canberra) 80 per cent will join the local Buteyko Supporters' Association (which now has more members than the local Asthma Foundation group).

On the last day, we also discuss the goals we want to achieve in the future and what to do if asthma symptoms should turn up again. Some people are already 100 per cent better; others who may be about 75 per cent symptom-free still need to make more progress and I let them know there will be follow-up sessions and more support available for anyone who needs it.

The progress you make depends on your commitment, the severity of your asthma and the drugs you have been taking. Asthma – as well as drug therapy – can impair the function of your adrenal system, and so your body needs time to repair itself.

There are some very active people who need to do very little after the workshop to maintain their normal breathing, but others need to go on working at it to keep up their best breathing. Some people like to pick a time every day – perhaps when they are watching the evening news on television – to check their breathing and practise their exercises for a few minutes.

Or, people may hit a stressful period in their lives, or experience an illness, and they may need to increase the practice of their exercises again for a while. We teach people to monitor their breathing daily and instruct them to continue to carry their medications with them and to use them when necessary.

As for Jessie, at the end of her Buteyko workshop, she didn't need her puffer any more. We were also able gradually to reduce the quantity of steroids she was taking, and she was weaned off them altogether over a period of a few months, with our GP's knowledge. She has been medication-free now for four years – and it has been the most enormous relief!

Angela, another physiotherapist, attended a Buteyko workshop in Scotland as an escort to her elderly mother who suffered from asthma:

My mother has always had a lot of chest complaints, beginning with pneumonia when she was 12 years old. That left her with weak lungs, and she went on to suffer from bronchitis. Her asthma started about 30 years ago, but it was sporadic. She would have a bout, and then recover. Then nine years ago she began taking salbutamol on a daily basis. Her asthma got progressively worse, deteriorating until she was put on steroid drugs.

Her health was such that she wasn't able to do much exercise. She couldn't do any heavy housework, or even walk up an incline. She couldn't establish a healthy sleeping pattern and she was two stone (nearly 13 kilos) overweight. Gradually, she was becoming disabled.

I first heard of the Buteyko method through a television programme and I offered to take her along to a workshop, every evening for a week. I went as her escort, on the basis that she is very shy and not good at going out by herself.

During that first session everything you have ever believed to be true about breathing is turned on its head. My mother – and other members of the group – sat looking a bit stunned and puzzled at first. But it was remarkable how quickly the techniques she was taught had an effect on her. It was immediately easier for her to breathe, while within two or three days she was able to tolerate my cats, which had always caused her an allergic reaction.

After the first evening of the workshop she took salbutamol on one occasion only. She did, however, continue with her steroid treatment, as recommended by the Buteyko practitioner, for another ten weeks. To get off all asthma drugs within the space of ten weeks is phenomenal for a lady in her seventies with long-term damage to her lungs.

One of the things that pleased her most was that she also lost a stone and a half (9.5 kilos) within that ten weeks – without making any effort to do so. She found that her appetite just melted away, and she followed instructions not to eat unless she felt hungry. It pleased her too that whereas she had always had a very pale, ashen face, she now has little rosy cheeks!

My mother's health is better across the board. She has no more hay fever, her energy levels are higher, her emotional state is better – and she can breathe without asthma symptoms. A lot of the problems which she had put down to her age have disappeared. She went to Blackpool Pier with her partner recently and for the first time in many years she was able to walk up an incline without intense effort and without losing her breath!

Jonathan, aged 32:

I used to have an asthma attack about once a week. I used an inhaler to relieve the symptoms, but I had to be careful in cold weather and after eating certain foods. Asthma runs in my family: my uncle died of an asthma attack.

I have found the Buteyko method to be very good. But you do have to work at it, and if you stop, you feel you need to start doing it again. I practise the breathing exercises twice a day for 10 to 15 minutes per session.

I've done a lot more sport since doing the Buteyko method, and I'm a lot fitter. I haven't had an asthma attack and I try to avoid using my inhaler completely. It's nine months since I did the workshop and I've used my inhaler only two or three times since then.

Sharon was ten years old when her mother took her to a Buteyko workshop:

I was concerned that at the age of ten Sharon was on salbutamol for her wheeziness. In the summer when she also had hay fever she was on steroids, too; one dose at night, another in the morning. I didn't want my daughter on these drugs, although the doctors assured me the dosage she was on would do her no harm, and yet I knew she needed some form of treatment. *

Then we signed up for a Buteyko workshop and it was great. I respected the fact that the practitioner told us not to stop her medication; it meant I didn't feel threatened or afraid of what they were doing. He stressed that we should keep on with steroids, which are 'preventers', but that we should only take one puff at a time of 'reliever' medicine (salbutamol). At the same time he explained to us how salbutamol made asthma worse by breaking breathing patterns. He said enough to make me feel that I didn't want my daughter to rely on this drug any more.

At the first session I was very excited but a bit bewildered. The practitioner gave us the background of Professor Buteyko in Russia and told us about the trial in Australia which had such positive results (see Appendix, page 177). He explained that we breathe incorrectly – and then he taught us some breath-holding exercises. We practised quiet, shallow breathing and learned how to measure our control pause [the major system for measuring breathing health, see page 75]. Sharon's control pause was ten at the start of the course – which means she was severely asthmatic – and we put it on the computer at home to encourage her. By the end of the week it was 40.

He also told us to be aware of our breathing, to close our mouths. He recommended we tape the mouth shut at night, and Sharon didn't seem to mind this at all. The feeling of the workshop was so positive; Sharon liked going along.

After a few days the practitioner talked to us about diet and recommended us to avoid milk and fish – and only to eat when hungry. Sharon was to have no chocolate or milk and we managed to stick to that.

For half an hour every night at bedtime during the course she practised her exercises, then control pause; then she repeated each one before taking her pulse. We practised the exercises every day, twice a day for a minimum of half an hour each time. It takes a bit of discipline to keep it up!

At the moment, some eight months after the course, Sharon has fewer symptoms of asthma and uses less salbutamol. She stopped using her puffer entirely for a while but this week has had to start again – so I'm keen to take up the exercises again with her.

Andrew, aged 40:

Although initially a bit sceptical, I have to confirm that after five days I do feel a lot better! It has made me aware of my breathing pattern, and also that I need to relax after my stressful job.

Today I walked three miles without being short of breath or even wheezing. I have stopped taking any medication, whereas I used to be on relievers and preventers. If anything it has also made me realise that I must not reach for my inhaler at the slightest sign of wheezing.

I am not saying that I am completely cured, but I do definitely feel a lot better than when I started this course. I would recommend this to anyone, whether they are asthmatic or not.

The Buteyko method, while especially suitable for people with asthma, can also help with a range of other disorders. Here, Marjorie Curtis describes how her symptoms of chronic fatigue disappeared after learning to retrain her breathing:

I have had Chronic Fatigue Syndrome (CFS) for about eight years. I've had every conventional and alternative medical test there is, and finally succeeded in getting a diagnosis five years ago. I've also tried dozens of remedies, both conventional and alternative, but none made any difference.

My symptoms included debilitating fatigue, aching bones and joints, poor concentration and memory, headaches, feeling too hot or too cold with night sweats, palpitations and weight gain. I also had nasal and throat mucus, visual disturbances, dry eyes, nightmares, breathlessness and sweating after the least physical exertion and mild sleep apnoea. In addition, my thyroid was underactive.

In 1995 I went to a Buteyko class. I was appalled by my pathetic results on the first day which were worse than some asthmatics in the group (I don't have asthma). But after just one week I felt better than I had for several years and my control pause was more than double what it was on my first day!

I have persisted with the daily exercises, three times a day for the first three months, and now twice a day. I continue to achieve longer control pauses. One of the best things about these exercises is that I am in control and – if I work hard – I will get the benefits.

The results have been amazing. I am much fitter now and no longer breathless. I can walk faster and even run – which I wasn't able to do for many years before I took the Buteyko course. I can also do heavy gardening and housework.

I am sleeping much better now and no longer feel exhausted when I wake up in the mornings. I sleep much less: between five and six hours each night, as I used to before I got CFS – although in the period before I took the Buteyko course I was sleeping 12 to 16 hours a night! I certainly no longer have 'sleep apnoea' – if I ever did.

I no longer need to sleep in the afternoons and I rarely have nightmares now. My GP has found that I need less thyroxine each day while I have lost more than 10 kilos since I did the course. I am less hungry and have lost my craving for sweet things.

The problem of mucus which used to bother me is much less and I can breathe easily at night. My heart palpitations have stopped since I learned the Buteyko method and I no longer suffer from temperature extremes.

I have recently felt well enough to take on professional work again because my mind is very much clearer than it has been for years. I feel really well now!

CHAPTER THREE

The Buteyko View of Asthma

In the last chapter we heard the stories of individuals whose health has been dramatically improved by practice of the Buteyko method. In this chapter we take a step back to look at why so many people have asthma today, what the medical profession has to offer them – and what Buteyko can offer instead.

Asthma on the rise

We've known about the disease we now call asthma for 4,000 years, yet modern medicine has so far failed to discover its causes – or to find a cure. Modern medical treatments are unsatisfactory, while doctors have little idea of how to prevent this disease. Yet statistics show a dramatic increase in asthma in the western world, painting a very worrying picture. Asthma

- is the only disease in the western world which is increasing to epidemic proportions.
- has for 40 years defeated modern medicine's attempts to reduce the number of deaths it causes.
- in children has doubled since the 1970s.

Surveys of UK schoolchildren conducted over the last ten years all point to the startling fact that in this country one child in eight now has asthma. An even higher proportion – one in five – has suffered from wheezing at some time in childhood. There are now some three million asthmatics in the UK. Every week around 40 people die from asthma in this country.

Yet in the 1960s there were just 100,000 people with asthma in the UK. In 1970, less than 4 per cent of children in the UK had asthma (or fewer than one in 25). So has the number of children with asthma really increased – or are we just better able to recognise the condition? Or, are we simply more inclined to call wheeziness 'asthma'?

Unfortunately, careful repeat studies point to a real increase in asthma. So why should this be? Various theories have been put forward to explain the rise in asthma, including air pollution, stress – and even the weather.

But while there is no doubt that pollution in our cities, particularly when combined with allergies, can trigger symptoms in people who already have asthma, there is no evidence that pollution **creates** more asthmatics. Indeed in the UK, the particles of soot and the dense sulphurous fumes which contributed to the infamous smogs of the 1950s have largely disappeared since the Clean Air Act – yet asthma has continued to rise. What's more, asthma is just as prevalent in the Scottish Highlands as it is in relatively smoggy urban areas.

So what about stress? Could this be causing increasing asthma? I believe it is a fallacy that we are under more stress today than were our ancestors, who struggled for survival against famine, plagues and wars. By contrast, we live relatively easy and protected lives. Of course stress can exacerbate asthma – whether you feel anger, depression, anxiety, joy or excitement – but stress itself cannot create asthma in the first place.

Some people have suggested that if asthma can be influenced by psychological events, asthmatics ought to have a readily identifiable type of personality. Over the years asthmatics have been described in a number of unflattering ways, ranging from irritable and fearful to complaining and obsessionally neurotic. But it strikes me as extremely unfair to blame a person who has a severe and frightening disease for being nervous and depressed, especially if you are going to treat them with drugs which will not eradicate their asthma.

As for the weather, in hot Israel, cold Canada, cool New Zealand and warm Australia, people still suffer from asthma. In America, which has all sorts of weather, 5,000 people die from asthma every year. Of course, some people with asthma feel better or worse in certain types of weather – but they still have asthma. Today, asthma is on the increase all over the globe.

What then is the reason or reasons for the phenomenal modern rise in the rates of asthma? The Buteyko method offers the following explanation.

- We have become obsessed with asthma. Doctors now try to diagnose it very early in children, often too early, so that illnesses previously called 'wheezy bronchitis' are now labelled asthma and treated accordingly. When you visit your doctor because of flu or a cold, he or she may well put you on asthma medications – 'just in case'. You start taking them and then, after a while, you discover that you now need them. You think you have developed asthma!

Probably the country most obsessed with asthma is Australia, where one in four children and one in ten adults are already diagnosed as having the disease. By the year 2020 medical authorities expect that one person in two will have asthma – and in a sadly self-fulfilling prophecy, so far it looks as if they are going to make it!

WHAT IS AN ASTHMA ATTACK?

An asthma attack happens when the tiny bronchotubes in your lungs become narrowed or constricted, making it difficult to breathe.

This constriction of the airways is caused by a combination of three factors:

- Bronchospasm, when the muscle rings around the airways contract.
- Swelling of the membranes of the airways, so that the air spaces are narrowed.
- An excess of mucus in the airways, secreted by the cells lining the bronchotubes.

An asthma attack is a vicious circle of hyperventilation, because as your airways narrow, spasm and become blocked by mucus, you feel an increasing need to breathe deeply. You may panic, gasping desperately for air. But the more you try to breathe deeply, the more your body's three defence mechanisms (above) work to make sure you don't increase your hyperventilation. The harder you try to breathe, the worse your asthma attack becomes – unless, using the Buteyko method, you learn to use techniques to bring your breathing under control.

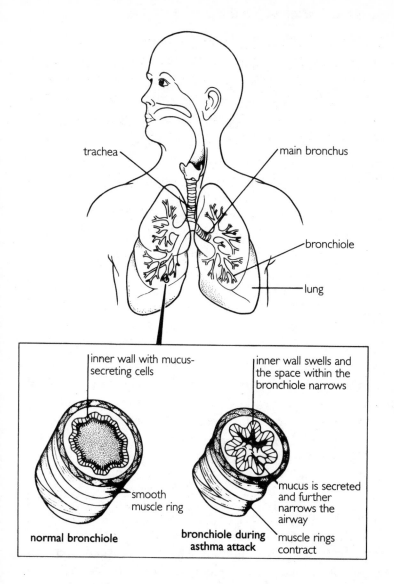

What happens during an asthma attack

Trying to make sense of asthma: the medical view

From a Buteyko point of view, modern medicine's attempts to classify asthma are not helpful. Traditionally, doctors have divided the disease into 'allergic' (extrinsic) and 'non-allergic' asthma. There are many people whose asthma is clearly triggered by allergic reactions, yet there are many others who have asthma attacks for a variety of reasons – some of them to do with allergy, but some not.

There is also another group of asthma sufferers who have no allergic problems, and they have been classified as having 'idiopathic' asthma. This sounds impressive, but in fact 'idiopathic' just means 'The disease is unique to the individual patient – or, in other words, 'We don't know the cause.'

Misunderstanding of the nature of asthma by conventional medicine has produced a complex division of asthma into different 'types'. If you wake up in the night unable to breathe you have 'nocturnal asthma'; if walking upstairs makes you breathless you have 'exercise-induced asthma'; if you get symptoms when you laugh it is 'emotional asthma' – and so on for 'occupational asthma'(your job), 'environmental asthma' (from pollution), 'aspirin asthma' (from taking aspirin) and 'self-induced' asthma – no doubt from crying about the injustice of having this confusing disease!

All this reminds me of the classification of animals in ancient China. The Chinese view was that there were 12 types of animal: those belonging to the Emperor, those which are small and jump, and so on, down to the final category, which comprised all animals not included in the previous groups!

However modern medicine tries to classify asthma, the clinical picture of an attack (see box on page 36) remains the same, whether it is induced by laughing or crying or sex or ice cream. And yet there is still no consensus amongst doctors, scientists and 'asthma educators' about the causes of asthma – or even about the causes of these different 'types' of asthma.

TRIGGER FACTORS, BUT NOT 'THE CAUSE' . . .

There are thousands of factors which can trigger an asthma attack, but modern medicine isolates six main trigger factors (as opposed to 'causes' of asthma):

- Exercise
- Viruses
- Infections
- Emotional factors, such as stress
- Allergies
- Drugs

Why modern medical treatments are unsatisfactory

Some 90 per cent of modern medical treatment for asthma involves prescription drugs. The other 10 per cent consists of advice on how to take the drugs properly, how to avoid trigger factors (see box) such as dust mites, how to maintain your best 'peak flow meter' readings (see page 103) and – sometimes – physiotherapy (see page 104). But in spite of these treatments, rates of asthma in the western world are getting worse, not better. Meanwhile, many people with asthma are suffering side effects from drug treatments.

It is also difficult or impossible to avoid many of the common trigger factors – such as atmospheric pollution or emotional upheaval – while peak flow meter readings are strangely resistant to all efforts to improve them. And from a Buteyko point of view, most physiotherapy only makes asthma worse.

The sad reality is that modern asthma treatments can go on for 20 years, 40 years, even 60 years. Meanwhile, dealing with asthma becomes a lifestyle, and asthma patients may well outlive their doctors – without ever finding a way to end the asthma which dominates their lives.

The fundamental problem with modern medical treatments is that they treat the symptoms of asthma – such as wheezing, coughing, phlegm and constriction of the airways – without tackling the cause. Yet in the words of Hippocrates two and a half thousand years ago, 'Not knowing the cause, the doctor has no right to treat the disease.'

To treat the cause of a disease is a very different matter

JOHN, AGED 72

I find I can control my wheezing! Taping my mouth has resulted in little mucus on my chest in the mornings, no headaches (after years of daily headaches) and no snoring. The control pause exercise works to clear my nose. I have more energy.

from treating the symptoms. Let's take, for example, the story of the plague and its treatment. This disease used to 'clean up' half of Europe rather as a snooker player 'cleans up' the table. At the time, many people considered it to be God's punishment for sin and they 'treated' themselves accordingly by going to church to pray (unless they were already infected, in which case they had to pray at home). They used other prophylactics too, like dressing in black and shouting, 'The Black Death is coming!'

But that was about all that people could do – until in 1882 Robert Koch discovered the real cause of the plague. It was not after all a punishment from God: it was instead a bacillus called *Yersina pestis*. Once the cause of the plague was understood, the cure for it – through vaccination – could be found.

The same is true of asthma – a breathing disorder. Once we understand the cause, we can do something about stopping it. Once we eliminate the cause, the problem will disappear.

If you can learn to normalise your breathing, you will not have asthma again, in spite of colds, playing sports, laughing, travelling, smoking or making love. There is only one thing you must not do: you must not overbreathe, or hyperventilate. If you do, you are breaking one of nature's most important laws, and asthma may return.

Asthma – breathing disorder

What makes Buteyko treatment crucially different from modern medical treatments is that it recognises that asthma is a **breathing disorder**, and so it sets out to investigate and change our breathing patterns.

Breathing is perhaps the most important function of our bodies. Every day we breathe in and out more than 20,000 times. We can survive for weeks without food, quite a few days without sleep and water – but only a few minutes without breathing. Yet even as we approach the end of the 20th century, most people's understanding of breathing is still very limited.

Until the second half of the 18th century, physicians believed that air was drawn into the lungs for the purpose of cooling the blood. Then the French chemist Antoine Lavoisier came up with his theory that oxygen was the 'gas of life' – as opposed to carbon dioxide, which was considered a 'waste gas' which we breathe out.

The logical conclusion seemed to be that we should all inhale more of the 'gas of life' in order to be healthy – and also exhale more 'waste gas'. Over the decades this idea has been promoted by physiotherapists, yoga teachers, doctors, sports coaches, army sergeants and aerobic instructors. **In the absence of even one scientific article to prove that deep breathing is good, it remains one of the great superstitions of the 20th century.**

However, there are hundreds of scientific studies which show that **overbreathing causes a range of health problems**, just as overeating, having high blood sugar, high blood pressure or high blood cholesterol can't be good for your health. For all of these essential aspects of health there are established norms, well known to the medical profession – except, strangely enough, breathing!

There is an internationally recognised norm for breathing too – although few doctors know of it. This is not the 'peak flow' measure used in conventional treatments for asthma, but a norm which depends (as the other norms do) on your age, height, gender and size. It is called the **minute volume,** and with the use of sophisticated equipment (available in some hospitals) it measures your lung ventilation in terms of the litres of air you breathe per minute.

A physiologically normal minute volume is between 4 and 6 litres of air per minute while you are at rest (less for children). People with asthma typically breathe two, three or four times that amount; **in other words, if you have asthma you are breathing enough for two, three or four people.** This is called **hyperventilation** – and, according to Buteyko, it is the major cause of asthma.

When you breathe, air passes from your windpipe (trachea) into your two main airways (bronchi). From there it

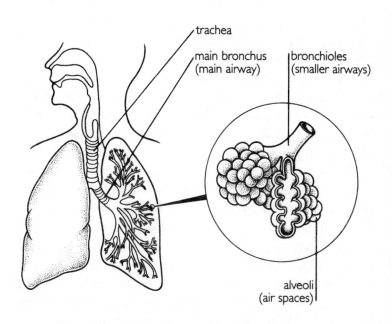

The structure of the lungs

goes through the small bronchioles to the tiny air sacs (alveoli) where oxygen is absorbed into your bloodstream. But then, far from going directly to the cells of our bodies, it goes through a complex chemical process called **respiration**.

Most oxygen molecules are carried in the blood by your red blood cells (although 5 per cent of it is dissolved in plasma, the colourless fluid that remains after red cells are filtered out of the blood). The material in red blood cells which 'grabs' and holds oxygen molecules is called **haemoglobin**, which combines with oxygen to make a new molecule called **oxyhaemoglobin**.

Once this oxygen-rich blood reaches the cells of the body which need it, the oxygen detaches itself from the red blood cell – to be used by the body's **metabolism** (the complex series of chemical reactions which transform fats, sugars and proteins into energy).

It is haemoglobin which makes it possible for your blood to carry the oxygen you need. Without it – and if oxygen were only dissolved in plasma – your heart would have to pump about 25 times as fast to deliver enough oxygen to your body cells.

Sometimes, however, haemoglobin can't release its oxygen to the body, and the heart starts pumping overtime. This is what happens to many asthmatics during an asthma attack: you feel a lack of oxygen so you desperately try to catch air, perhaps opening the windows in an attempt to get more oxygen. Yet despite breathing rapidly, often through the mouth, it doesn't seem to help.

Why should this be? Surely – we have been led to believe – deep breathing gives us more oxygen.

But this is the paradox which lies at the heart of under-

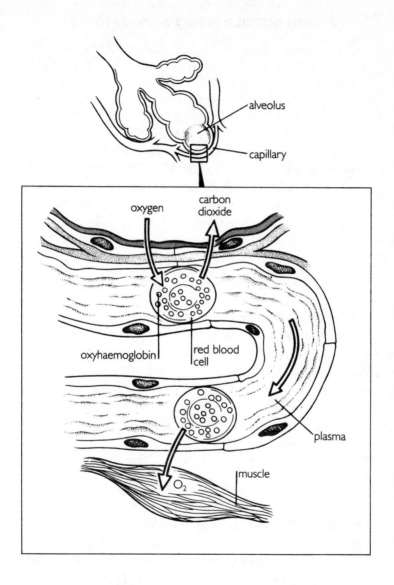

An oxygen molecule's journey to the bloodstream

CARBON DIOXIDE IS NOT A 'WASTE GAS'!

Lavoisier in the second part of the 18th century gave the name oxygen to what has since been thought of as 'the gas of life'. By contrast, carbon dioxide, which was shown to kill mice at high concentrations, was believed to be a poisonous, or at best, a 'waste' gas. Yet a later experiment with baby mice, which were put in a container with pure oxygen, showed that this 'gas of life' made them blind. For some reason not many people know about this experiment.

The common – but false – assumption that after inhaling oxygen we exhale a 'waste gas' called carbon dioxide (CO_2) has led to a fundamental misunderstanding of asthma. In fact carbon dioxide is one of the most important chemical regulators of the human body, monitoring the activity of the heart, the blood vessels and the respiratory system.

- The rate and depth of our breathing is regulated by the amount of carbon dioxide in our blood, as Haldane discovered in 1905.
- When carbon dioxide is removed from the body in undue quantities by excessive artificial ventilation of the lungs, the heart and circulation gradually fail and death results (as Professor Yandell Henderson of Yale discovered in 1909).
- The level of oxygen in the room where you are reading this book is 20 per cent – the normal level of this gas in

standing the Buteyko method: the truth is that **when you overbreathe** (i.e. breathe more than the physiological norm) **you are actually getting less oxygen, not more.** This is because our bodies need to maintain a certain level of carbon dioxide in the blood in order for our haemoglobin our atmosphere. You would probably not notice if the oxygen level doubled or even tripled around you because our bodies are 'blind' to higher levels of oxygen. And if the oxygen level dropped considerably, you would be unlikely to notice any difference in your breathing. Only if the level dropped below 15 per cent – as it does at high altitudes – would you be aware of the difference.

Contrast the situation with carbon dioxide. Asthmatics have between 3.5 and 4.5 per cent of carbon dioxide in their alveolar air. If this were to be decreased by as little as 0.1 per cent anyone – whether they were asthmatic or not – would develop dizziness, palpitations, wheezing, a blocked nose – or a mild asthma attack.

These figures indicate that our bodies are 50 times more sensitive to changes in carbon dioxide levels than they are to changes in oxygen levels. It follows that carbon dioxide is far more important to your body than oxygen.

- If an asthmatic can 'normalise' his or her carbon dioxide level by raising it to 5.5 or 6 per cent, he or she can get rid of their asthma. Experiments have shown that more than 10 per cent of carbon dioxide causes loss of consciousness, but there is never any need to increase carbon dioxide to such an extent, and the Buteyko method certainly does not involve raising carbon dioxide levels above normal.

to release the oxygen which we so desperately need.

When we overbreathe, we are upsetting the delicate balance between carbon dioxide and oxygen in our bloodstreams that we need to maintain in order to make use of the oxygen in our body cells. Yes, we are breathing in more

A PIONEERING STUDY OF BREATHING

One of history's great investigators into breathing was John Haldane, an Englishman who lived between 1860 and 1936. He developed methods which enabled scientists to learn how much oxygen and carbon dioxide are contained in a person's blood and lungs at any time, and how our bodies regulate breathing in response to these substances. Haldane also studied the breathing process and the amounts of energy that our bodies use in order to breathe.

Haldane's work has helped us to understand the fundamental principles of human breathing, so that by the mid-20th century it was established that oxygen passes into our bloodstreams through the thin membrane of the alveoli without having to be 'pumped' by any other

oxygen, but we are also breathing out more carbon dioxide – and without the carbon dioxide we can't 'use' the oxygen.

This paradoxical fact is explained in a physiological law called the Verigo-Bohr effect, which states that when levels of carbon dioxide in the blood are lowered, the chemical bond between oxygen and haemoglobin increases. Because haemoglobin won't 'let go' of its oxygen, this makes it hard for the cells of the brain, heart and kidneys to get the oxygen they need. The consequence is that the deeper you breathe, the less oxygen your body cells will get. We know the results of this kind of over-breathing as **hyperventilation. One of Professor Buteyko's most fascinating discoveries was that all asthmatics over-breathe – and that the rate of this overbreathing increases during asthma attacks.**

process. It was Haldane, too, who established the importance of the right quantities of carbon dioxide in our breathing by the techniques he invented of sampling the gas in the alveoli.

Haldane's book *Respiration* (1936) with its analysis of alveolar air influenced many scientists – in particular, the medical student Konstantin Buteyko.

Ultimately Haldane became involved in secret research for the British Navy into the control of oxygen and carbon dioxide in damaged submarines. Many of his findings are still classified as 'top secret'. Unfortunately, he was not interested in asthma, which in his day was not considered a fatal disease. Yet his work helped us to understand that the process we call **respiration** is not just a matter of inhaling oxygen and exhaling carbon dioxide.

Hyperventilation

Most of us know from experience what happens when we breathe 'too much', perhaps when we are blowing up balloons or blowing on the fire: we feel dizzy, we may have palpitations and if we keep at it we may get chest pains and even lose consciousness. This is **hyperventilation**, another name for 'overbreathing', and it was first described in 1870 by a Dr Da Costa who called it the 'soldiers' heart' syndrome – because he noticed how it caused 'disabling shortness of breath and irritable heart' in soldiers during the American Civil War.

Modern medical and scientific texts have many conflicting definitions of hyperventilation, but from a Buteyko point of view the key to understanding the term lies in the word itself. 'Hyper' means too much, while 'ventilation' refers to lung ventilation. If you measure the ventilation of your lungs, compare it to the established norms and find you are above the norms (usually 4 to 6 litres of air per minute), then you are hyperventilating.

Medical misunderstanding of hyperventilation is related to the extraordinary fact that most asthma specialists don't know what the norms of lung ventilation should be. This means that the doctors who treat breathing disorders don't know what it is to have truly healthy breathing. They argue that this doesn't matter and that you should 'leave it to your body'. Yet if you went to a diabetes specialist asking what your blood sugar level should be, he or she would never say, 'It doesn't matter; leave it to your body. Oh, and take this and this medicine three times a day...'

Some doctors also argue that rather than hyperventilation causing asthma (the Buteyko view), asthma attacks **induce** hyperventilation as the body's natural reaction to lack of oxygen. However, the first trial to measure lung ventilation in the western world (which took place at the Mater Hospital, Australia in 1994–5 – see Appendix, page 177) proved that all asthmatics hyperventilate even when they are not having asthma attacks. To the considerable surprise of many scientists, all 39 asthmatics in the trial had an average intake of 15 litres of air per minute, three times the norm.

What's more, that same trial demonstrated that patients who learned the Buteyko method decreased their hyperventilation from 15 litres per minute to 9 litres per minute. As a result of that decrease they were able comfortably to reduce their usage of bronchodilator drugs by 90 per cent, and of steroid drugs by 50 per cent.

The 'control' group which did not use the Buteyko method and did not decrease lung ventilation showed no improvement.

Unfortunately, modern medicine recognises only acute, visible hyperventilation, usually caused by anxiety, but these cases represent a mere 5 per cent of the total. The other 95 per cent of people who hyperventilate – with a broad range of slowly developing and cumulative symptoms – are left without treatment.

We have seen how efficient control of our bodies' metabolism depends on maintaining a delicate balance

---

DEEP BREATHING TEST

You may want to try this test yourself, although beware: it may provoke an asthma attack or, if you are epileptic, a fit.

- Sit down and start to breathe fast and deeply through your mouth, as you do when you are running.
- Within 30–40 seconds (far less for some people) you will develop unpleasant symptoms which may include dizziness, palpitations, rising blood pressure, coughing and wheezing. (Don't keep this up for long: if you were to keep going you could develop a serious headache, migraine, asthma attack – or you could black out.)
- When you develop these initial symptoms, stop breathing deeply, close your mouth and try to breathe gently through your nose. Your symptoms will go away.
- If you try the test again, you will develop the symptoms again.

The point of this test is that these symptoms are caused not by too much oxygen, but by too little carbon dioxide.

---

between oxygen and carbon dioxide in our bloodstreams. When we breathe at the appropriate depth and rate – more during exercise, less when we are relaxing – this balance is undisturbed. But when we overbreathe, our levels of carbon dioxide drop dramatically.

Most of us think of the need for oxygen as the key to our breathing, but in fact the level of carbon dioxide is the 'marker' which determines the rate at which we should breathe. The paradox is that while you are taking in more oxygen by overbreathing, that oxygen isn't getting to where it is needed in your body and brain. This is because lack of carbon dioxide causes constriction of the blood vessels, reducing blood supply to the brain and to the rest of the body.

When carbon dioxide levels in the blood go down, so does the acid content of the blood, causing a phenomenon

---

ASTHMA AND HEADACHES

You may have noticed that during an asthma attack, or when you are coughing, or after using bronchodilators, you feel dizzy or develop a headache. This is sometimes considered an insignificant side effect of bronchodilators.

Buteyko, however, explains that your headache is a result of hyperventilation, to which you are especially prone after a sustained cough or severe asthma attack. What is happening is that lack of carbon dioxide is causing narrowing of the blood vessels in your brain. For the same reason, your heart will be pumping hard, you may be having chest pains or even a heart attack.

Far from being a side effect of asthma drugs, these are the classic symptoms of hyperventilation.

known as 'alkaline blood'. When the acid/alkaline balance of your blood is upset, the results can include bronchospasm, suppression of the immune system in general and the development of allergic reactions in particular, overproduction of mucus, disturbance of the nervous system, loss of oxygenation and imbalance of the metabolic processes in the bronchial cells – or, in other words, asthma.

So, to sum up, when you hyperventilate, not only does less blood get to important areas of your body, but the oxygen carried by the blood is less easily released there and the low levels of carbon dioxide in the body lead directly to asthma symptoms.

In 1909 Professor Yandell Henderson conducted an experiment on a number of perfectly healthy dogs. He put them on breathing machines which forced them to hyperventilate. They soon started to tremble, as asthmatics do after a dose of nebuliser, and within four to six hours, in spite of having 'plenty of air', all of them were dead.

In 1952, Professor Buteyko discovered that **hyper-**

**HYPERVENTILATION AND ASTHMA –
A SUMMARY**

- Asthma attacks happen when you increase your rate of overbreathing, or hyperventilation.
- If you know how to control your hyperventilation, you can overcome an asthma attack.
- If you 'normalise' your breathing you can cure your asthma.
- You can't cure asthma without normalising your breathing.

ventilation is a major cause of asthma. He argued that this is not merely a 'trigger factor' because all asthmatics hyperventilate, whether their asthma is classified as 'emotional', mild, severe, stress-related, occupational or triggered by an infection.

Professor Buteyko also found that all asthmatics recover from asthma when they stop hyperventilating, because when you normalise your breathing you also eliminate bronchospasm, inflammation and mucus from the lungs.

The next time you have an asthma attack – or symptoms such as wheezing or tightness in the chest – take a look at your breathing. You will find that it is much deeper than usual.

Hyperventilation – the missing link

It makes interesting reading to research how close scientists of the past have been to cracking the asthma puzzle – and to making the link between hyperventilation and a range of other diseases.

Some scientists have been very near to Professor Buteyko's discovery that hyperventilation is the cause of many illnesses. Some have tried to understand the powerful effect of carbon dioxide on the body, but there has been too big a gap between their thinking and that of doctors, who have traditionally regarded carbon dioxide as a 'waste gas' and who have relied heavily on drugs to treat their patients.

Laennec (who invented the stethoscope in the first half of the 19th century) was closer to the Buteyko method and to the solution of the asthma puzzle than many modern scientists. He concluded that asthma was caused by spasms of the bronchial muscles, and that if the asthmatic held his breath he could breathe naturally for one or two breaths after that, clearly demonstrating that bronchospasm was capable of momentary relaxation. He was very close to understanding that the human body – a very sophisticated chemical factory – is often able to produce the necessary chemicals to heal itself without resorting to the help of drugs.

Today's doctors recognise that by deliberate hyperventilation and overbreathing asthmatics can produce asthma attacks, or make their asthma worse. They may put this down to 'drying out the airways' or 'cooling the airways' (see page 113), while Buteyko practitioners would say it was lack of carbon dioxide, but what is interesting is that they have never tried to prevent asthma by deliberately **decreasing** hyperventilation.

The articles of Dr D. Innocenti (in *A Textbook for Physiotherapists*) on chronic hyperventilation syndrome are 15 years old now, yet many of his observations are not accepted by today's doctors. 'Hyperventilation has been recognised for many generations as an acute disorder,' he wrote, but 'unfortunately, the Chronic Habitual Hyperventilation Syndrome more frequently goes unrecognised.

DOROTHY, AGED 44

My breathing has much improved during the week of the workshop. I have taken no salbutamol since Sunday. Despite being in the presence of a known trigger – cats – I did not get wheezy. My chest feels tight but not wheezy. My appetite has decreased.

Chronic hyperventilators may be referred to a succession of specialists who find no evidence of organic disease. Many become chronic invalids with gross anxiety neuroses as a result of the continuance of undiagnosed, alarming symptoms. The situation is self-perpetuating in this group of people who breathe in such a manner that their arterial carbon dioxide level is persistently low; and this may be the basis of a variety of symptoms.'

Dr Innocenti gives this table of some of the symptoms of chronic hyperventilation:

- Cardiovascular symptoms: palpitation, tachycardia, peripheral vasoconstriction.
- Respiratory symptoms: bronchospasm, breathlessness, air hunger, excessive sighing, chest pain.
- Neurological symptoms: paraesthesia, dizziness, lack of co-ordination, disturbance of vision, disturbance of hearing, black-outs.
- Musculoskeletal symptoms: muscle pains, involuntary contractions, tremors, cramps, tetany.
- General symptoms: exhaustion, lethargy, weakness, sleep disturbance, headache, disturbance of concentration and memory, anxiety, panic attacks, phobic states, excessive sweating.

According to Professor Buteyko, these are just one tenth of all the symptoms of chronic hyperventilation, which he believes may cause headaches, migraine, chronic fatigue, schizophrenia – and of course, asthma – to name but a few.

There is a link between hyperventilation and cystic fibrosis, too, in which patients suffer from having very sticky mucus in their lungs. There is a further interesting link between asthma and epilepsy in that in both of these disorders, hyperventilation is a major cause of attacks or fits.

According to Anthony Hopkins in his book *Epilepsy*, 'one proposed mechanism for the association between stress and seizures is hyperventilation. Matson and colleagues reported three patients who, when anxious, tended to hyperventilate unconsciously. At these times, EEG and clinical seizure activity increased, correlating with a reduction in alveolar $P CO_2$. The hypothesis that anxiety leads to hyperventilation and, by lowering $P CO_2$ triggers the seizure activity, was supported by their observation that administration of 5% carbon dioxide could prevent or terminate the seizure activity, even though anxiety and overbreathing continued.'

The fact is that epileptics – like asthmatics and people with a range of other related disorders – always hyperventilate. With reconditioning of their breathing patterns through the Buteyko technique, to establish proper levels of carbon dioxide, it is possible to prevent seizures – and asthma attacks – without the use of drugs.

An overbreathing society

There are a variety of reasons why we develop hyperventilation, or habitual overbreathing, including infections, stress and medications. But perhaps the most important reason is that we are **trained** to overbreathe – and we have the habit of overbreathing. Look at the people around you: as they walk down the street, nearly all of them breathe through their mouths, an orifice which is bigger than the nose and which takes in far more air. Look at children, too: their mouths are open.

Western culture teaches that 'deep breathing' is good for us. When I ask patients where they got this idea, they say, 'It's common knowledge' or 'I was brought up to believe this' or 'That's what the doctor said.' Yet this belief has caused no end of problems. Just as we first dislike alcohol when we first try it, but overcome our dislike to develop a 'taste' for it, so we can learn to develop a 'taste' for deep breathing.

If you are taught to breathe deeply, you can override the delicate reflex in your respiratory centre, a group of cells located in the medulla of the brain which is responsible for the regulation of breathing. Your respiratory centre then becomes adjusted to a lower level of carbon dioxide and you feel that this is 'normal' breathing.

To take another analogy, some dancers and models have a culture of good posture. They need it and so they have cultivated it. The rest of us don't need it and so we don't care about our bad posture. Instead, we visit chiropractors to treat the symptoms of our back pain, and our chiropractors don't mind at all when we come to see them again and again! But visiting a chiropractor will not make your posture better: this is something you have to do for yourself.

It follows that with asthma, medical treatments which address the symptoms will do nothing to change the cause of asthma. There is no medication in existence which can normalise your breathing patterns for you. The Buteyko method, however, can teach you how to normalise your breathing, putting an end to asthma symptoms and the need for medication.

Learning to breathe again

Professor Buteyko teaches that it is possible to re-learn correct breathing. Some doctors say that this is impossible because breathing is an involuntary process, so that even if asthmatics do hyperventilate, there is nothing you can do about that.

It is true that many of our bodily mechanisms – including breathing – are controlled by 'automatic' chemical and physical means. But breathing can **also** respond to our voluntary control. For example, we can hold our breath when swimming under water, or we can increase our rate of breathing when we blow up balloons.

We all know too that there are other 'non-automatic' factors which can cause us to breathe more, including emotion and stress. Another of these factors is habit.

The Buteyko method teaches us to overcome this habit, to retrain our breathing centres, and to 'reset' our level of breathing to normal levels – with tremendous positive implications for our health in general, and for asthma in particular.

The 'advancing edge of research'

Doctors admit that the present trend of increasing prevalence of asthma and allergic disorders shows no early signs of reversing, which suggests that those who research the causes of asthma will not lack work for decades to come. Doctors also admit that there is still a good deal of doubt about the mechanisms that cause asthma, especially in the minority of people who do not have 'allergic' asthma.

Yet still, at intervals, they proclaim new departures in

asthma research, like the prospect of genetic engineering. This, however, remains many decades away. Meanwhile, the leading edge of research shows that non-allergic asthma patients have a larger number of 'helper T lymphocytes' than others. Might it not be possible, speculate asthma researchers, to treat asthma by attacking these 'helper T cells' – perhaps with other powerful drugs?

But from a Buteyko point of view, what we should be asking is – what effect is such a drug going to have on hyperventilation? If it decreases hyperventilation, it could be a cure for asthma (providing it does not have major side effects). If it does not, it will increase hyperventilation, and will eventually cause more harm to asthma sufferers than other, less powerful drugs.

The truth is there is no 'magic pill' which can cure asthma, now or in the future. The cause of asthma is hyperventilation, and so the best way to prevent it is to retrain your breathing using the Buteyko method.

CHAPTER FOUR

You and Your Asthma

Now that we have explained the scientific basis of the Buteyko approach to asthma, we can return to the practical questions of what you can do about your own over-breathing. In this chapter we see why asthma is in fact your body's way of defending you against hyperventilation. Between 20 and 30 per cent of people have a genetic predisposition which makes them react to overbreathing with spasms of the bronchotubes. If you have asthma, you are one of those people – but you can work with your body (not against it) to prevent this problem on a day-to-day basis.

Asthma as a defence mechanism

Your body has many defence mechanisms to protect it from harm. For instance, when you hit your head against a wall, you feel pain – which tells you to stop. Pain is the message from your body which stops you going on hurting yourself, and as such, it is not a bad thing.

But suppose you respond to your pain by taking painkillers. You get a bit of relief at first, but if you keep hitting your head on that wall, you will need stronger and ever stronger painkillers. In the long run – because you are treating the symptoms and not the cause – you will end up not only with a serious headache, but with side effects from the drugs you have taken. Your 'treatment' has not been a success!

This may seem like a silly analogy, but in fact it has many parallels with medical treatments for asthma. Modern asthma drugs treat the symptoms of asthma, but not the cause. Meanwhile, we ignore the message of asthma which, like pain, is one of our body's natural defence mechanisms – because asthma is essentially your body's way of helping to restrict the amount of air you are breathing.

When you overbreathe – and, as we have seen, you may be breathing at three or four times the healthy rate – the level of carbon dioxide in your body goes down (because you are breathing out too much carbon dioxide). In order to survive, we need to maintain a carbon dioxide level of between 3 and 6.5 per cent. If you overbreathe too much for too long, your carbon dioxide level will sink below 3 per cent and you will die. It is asthma which saves you from this fate.

Asthma is the message your body is sending you to stop overbreathing. It makes you wheeze, constricts your bronchotubes, makes extra mucus, decreases your lung capacity – all in the attempt to stop you breathing out so much carbon dioxide. The symptoms we experienced in the Deep Breathing Test – showing the effects of hyperventilation, such as dizziness, blocked nose, palpitations and so on – are likely to occur too.

Unfortunately, conventional treatments ensure that you override the message of asthma. You are given

---

KATE, AGED 29

I have not taken any salbutamol since the start of the Buteyko course, and I have not needed to. I am really delighted with my progress and hope to consult my doctor about stopping my steroids. I will certainly tell him about the Buteyko method; I can hardly believe that in these few days I have rid myself of asthma.

---

bronchodilators to open up your airways – and when your body sends you an even stronger message with a stronger asthma attack, you are given stronger bronchodilators to combat the constriction in your chest. These drugs act against your body's own defense mechanism, making it possible for you to exhale even more carbon dioxide – and so your asthma gets worse.

Once you understand the meaning of these unquestionably unpleasant symptoms they can become your friends, because they are giving you some very important information – that you are overbreathing. If you respond to the language of your body by decreasing your breathing to end hyperventilation, the message is not needed any more and the symptoms will disappear.

Asthma will go away if you stop overbreathing, just as pain will go away if you stop banging your head against a wall. So listen to that message – and don't shoot the messenger!

A day in the life of your asthma – before learning the Buteyko method

Despite these warnings, you have probably been trying to

'beat' your asthma with one or more of the range of prescription asthma drugs. But 'beating' your asthma means 'beating' your body – because asthma is your body's own defence mechanism against overbreathing.

So 'if you can't beat them, join them'. I suggest that you start by investigating your asthma, to understand how you breathe throughout the day.

Let's start now. Say it is evening while you are reading this page...

In the evening...

While you are reading this page,

- **Do keep your mouth closed.** This is especially relevant to some elderly people who have the habit of using their lips when reading. If you can, hold the book above your face. Professor Buteyko has observed that looking down increases your breathing (we don't know why, although this could be a reflex) and in addition your eyes will get tired much sooner.
- **Don't lie down** unless you are really sleepy, because lying down will also increase your breathing. (This is because we are naturally upright creatures; just try doing a headstand for a few minutes and you will feel the effects on your body of not being upright!) Stay sitting upright in a chair to read, watch television, think or meditate. Use your bed only for sleep and avoid taking sleeping pills. It's best only to go to bed when you feel really sleepy: if insomnia is a problem, the Buteyko method will solve this for you too.
- **Don't forget to take your steroids** if you had any

asthma problems today. You don't yet know the Buteyko method, which will decrease your breathing, and so steroids are the best drugs to reduce your breathing artificially in the meantime and to prevent asthma attacks.

- **Don't take a bronchodilator to 'prevent' asthma.** This is not a preventive medicine. On the contrary, bronchodilator drugs will expand your bronchotubes for a few hours, increasing hyperventilation. This means that your body will have to produce phlegm to decrease the resulting loss of carbon dioxide. When – as morning approaches – the bronchodilating effects of the drugs you have taken wear off, you will suffer bronchoconstriction again – and a lot of phlegm as well.

- **Don't go to bed if your asthma is bad.** Fix it first with steroids to prevent night-time problems. If you don't do this, asthma will wake you up anyway, as the small asthma problems of the day become major problems during the night.

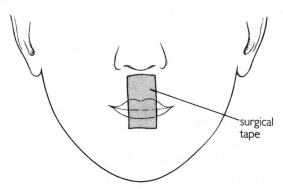

surgical tape

Taping your mouth helps you check what is going on while you are asleep

- **Do make sure your mouth is closed when you go to bed.** As we have seen, breathing through the mouth adds to overbreathing. If necessary, use a micropore surgical tape to keep it shut – and to check what is going on while you are asleep. If you wake up in the morning and the tape is still in place, you may not need to tape your mouth again. But if the tape is not there, it means that you opened your mouth in your sleep and for at least a few hours you have been hyperventilating, losing precious carbon dioxide.

  Some people develop a kind of claustrophobia when their mouths are taped, and if you feel anxious about it, tape your mouth for a while before you go to bed – and watch television for a bit – so that you can get used to it and feel sure that you are able to breathe through your nose.

  If it is your child who has asthma, try to explain to your child why you want to put tape across his or her mouth. If your child can't accept the idea, wait until he or she is asleep and then gently shut his mouth and put the tape across.

  Don't worry that your child is going to suffocate because of the tape; if he feels he is not getting enough air, he can take the tape off very easily.

  Thousands of mothers around the world have tried this method without making any complaint about it. But if you are still worried, sit beside your child for a while while he sleeps. You will see in the morning that he feels much better after a night in which his mouth was closed – because overbreathing causes far more harm than attempts to normalise it.

- **Do sleep on your left side.** Professor Buteyko discovered experimentally that this reduces hyperventilation. If your asthma is still bad and you want to sleep, then try to sleep on a chair. This certainly helps, as many severe asthmatics have discovered, because you are in an upright position.

- **Do check your asthmatic child two or three times during the night.** If he has turned over on to his back, turn him on to his side again. If his mouth is open, close it. If his breathing is heavy and wheezy, shake him to 'shake off' the hyperventilation and break the pattern of deep breathing.
- **Do set your alarm clock to break up your sleep if you have asthma attacks in the night.** Try to wake up about one hour before you expect an asthma attack and sit upright. This will help to prevent night-time attacks.

In the morning...

- **Do get up straight away and try to control your breathing.**
- **Do breathe only through your nose.**
- **Do avoid milk at breakfast time** (and indeed any time). Use juice on your cereal instead. Professor Buteyko believes that milk is not necessary to our diet and can be harmful (though a few drops in a cup of tea won't make much difference if you really feel you can't start the day without it). **If you are not hungry, don't eat breakfast.** If you are, don't overeat because overeating increases hyperventilation.
- **Do try not to cough.** If possible, suppress your cough

UNDERSTANDING THE PROBLEM IS THE FIRST STEP TOWARDS THE SOLUTION

Even before you start to learn the Buteyko method, you can investigate and get to know your own breathing – and your own asthma:

- Sit down, relax and start listening to your breathing, in and out.
- How do you **feel** your breath? As a movement of air in your nose? A cooling sensation in your nostrils? Or as a movement in your chest, abdomen or head? It doesn't matter how or where you feel your breathing, as long as you can 'hear' it and be aware of it.
- Spend as much time as you need to achieve a clear awareness of your breathing; 10 to 15 minutes will probably be enough.
- Memorise your breathing pattern at rest when you don't have obvious asthma problems.
- For three days, listen to your asthma in different circumstances, i.e.
    – in the morning

or cough very gently with your mouth closed. Coughing is in itself a form of hyperventilation, while hanging on to phlegm is part of your lungs' defence mechanism. Coughing on top of a wheeze will lead to an asthma attack.

- **Do use a bronchodilator if – but only if – you feel tightness in your chest.** You don't yet know the Buteyko method, so use one puff – preferably of Ventolin, because it gives a much lower dose than most other bronchodilators. Only use bronchodilators when you

- during sport
- during lunch
- during an asthma attack, or just a wheeze
- during a cough or tightness of the chest
- after using bronchodilators
- before and after using your peak flow meter
- during conversation
- when you have a blocked nose or palpitations or a headache
- while you are walking and/or going upstairs
- before and after dinner
- before bed

Be attentive and you will discover many interesting things:

- You will be able to connect different aspects of your breathing with the stages of your asthma.
- You will learn that it is impossible to have an asthma attack unless your breathing is deep.
- You will learn what happens to your breathing when you wake up in the morning because of an asthma attack.

really need them – and as little as possible. If you decrease your dose of bronchodilator, you are taking the first step towards having fewer problems with asthma.

- **Do keep taking your steroids for the time being.** Until you learn the Buteyko method, it is safer to stay on steroids which artificially decrease your breathing.
- **Do not use your peak flow meter.** This may produce bronchospasm, which shows itself as wheezing or coughing (see page 103).

During the day...

- **Do keep your mouth closed for breathing** – whether you go out to work or stay at home all day. Remind yourself at intervals; it is important to develop the habit of breathing through your nose to reduce hyperventilation.
- **Do take your steroids now if you forgot them in the morning.** Try never to forget your steroids; far better to forget your bronchodilator – forever.
- **Do breathe through your nose all day long,** whether you are walking, driving, eating, working, resting or playing sport.
- **Do check your control pause** (see page 75) from time to time, instead of using your peak flow meter. That way you will become familiar with what is happening to your breathing throughout the day, whatever you are doing.
- **Do count how many puffs of bronchodilator you have taken** – and congratulate yourself if you took fewer than usual.

So far, this is not the Buteyko method. It is just common sense.

CHAPTER FIVE

A Buteyko Workshop

Earlier chapters in this book have looked at both the theory and personal experience of getting better from asthma. This chapter moves on to describe the process of a Buteyko workshop from the practitioner's point of view.

Learning the Buteyko method

As we have seen in Chapter Two, during a Buteyko workshop, patients learn to recognise their overbreathing patterns and – through breathing exercises – to retrain and recondition their breathing to normal levels. The programme includes education about the effects of lifestyle and behaviour on breathing, and the causes of hyperventilation are addressed.

The Buteyko method takes discipline – and, yes, it does take time to learn. It is sometimes quite difficult for adults at first, because they have a lifetime of bad breathing habits to overcome, but they soon master it when they realise what excellent results come from a little effort. And the good news is that it easy for children. Children from four years can do it for themselves, and there is a special programme which enables parents to help their babies learn

BUTEYKO EXPLAINS WHAT SEEM TO BE PARADOXES

Q. Why is it easier for asthmatics to breathe in than to breathe out?

A. Because your defence mechanism, bronchoconstriction, works only when you exhale – because it is designed to stop you losing carbon dioxide.

Q. Why in clean New Zealand or West Germany is the death rate from asthma higher than in polluted Romania or East Germany?

A. Because treatment of asthma in developed countries involves the use of more powerful bronchodilator drugs, including nebulisers for home use.

Q. Why do former sportsmen often suffer terrible disorders when they retire from sport?

A. Because nearly all of them developed serious hyperventilation while they played sport, but at that time they compensated for it by physical exercise, during which the body produces carbon dioxide. After they quit sport, however, they stop exercising to the same extent – and stop making extra carbon dioxide – but continue hyperventilating, which causes severe illnesses and ultimately death.

normal breathing patterns. Children of five and over get results more quickly than adults, no matter how severe their asthma. It is important that the Buteyko method should be taught only by a certified Buteyko practitioner, so do ask to see credentials (a diploma or certificate from Professor Buteyko). The method is taught either in groups or on a one-to-one basis.

Q. Why do we develop a 'second wind' while taking exercise?

A. During exercise, breathing becomes fast and deep and your level of carbon dioxide goes down, creating a lack of oxygen in the muscles which makes you feel tired. But if you have the willpower to continue exercising, your level of carbon dioxide starts to grow, 'sped up' by intensive muscle work which makes carbon dioxide. Your carbon dioxide level is raised higher than when you started and the 'respiratory centre' in your brain is adjusted to this. When your carbon dioxide level goes up, the oxygenation of your body improves and oxygen goes into your muscle cells so that you no longer feel breathless or tired: you get a 'second wind'. (See Chapter Seven.)

Q. Why does asthma often become significantly worse after smokers give up cigarettes?

A. Because asthmatics are under stress when they give up smoking and so they hyperventilate. Some people even develop asthma when they give up smoking. Yet we all know that smoking is bad for our health: fewer people know that nicotine affects your breathing centre and increases hyperventilation. So the trick is to quit smoking without putting yourself under too much stress as a result!

Workshop: day one

During the first session you are asked to fill in various forms so that the practitioner is aware of what asthma medications you are using and of the steroids you have taken – or ceased to take. The practitioner will also want to know about any other illnesses you have, any recent severe asthma attacks, hospital admissions, respiratory arrests or clinical deaths. Children under the age of 16 must be accompanied by one or both parents.

Then the Buteyko practitioner explains the essence of the Buteyko discovery, which is that overbreathing is the cause of asthma. He will ask the workshop to try the Deep Breathing Test (see page 51). This demonstrates that too little carbon dioxide – not too much oxygen – is the cause of the unpleasant symptoms of hyperventilation, such as dizziness, coughing, wheezing and palpitations.

Next, the Buteyko practitioner explains how to measure your own breathing pattern using the **control pause** (see box). The relationship between your control pause, carbon dioxide levels, breathing and asthma is explained.

The practitioner explains that carbon dioxide is a natural bronchodilator, or 'natural salbutamol', and also talks about issues such as the Verigo-Bohr effect (which shows that our bodies need carbon dioxide in order to make use of oxygen, see page 48) and the impact of carbon dioxide on the acid-alkali balance of your blood (see page 52).

Then the practitioner explains asthma as one of the symptoms of hyperventilation and describes how your body reacts to the loss of carbon dioxide (which follows overbreathing) by activating a range of defence mechanisms, from mucus production to constriction of the bronchotubes.

A discussion of asthma medication follows, during which the practitioner makes sure that everybody understands the difference between 'relievers' (bronchodilators such as salbutamol) and 'preventers' (steroids such as

THE CONTROL PAUSE – THE MAJOR SYSTEM FOR MEASURING BREATHING HEALTH

To measure your control pause, sit comfortably in an upright chair, relax and breathe out. Then breathe in normally and out again, holding your nose after the outbreath. Count the seconds using a stopwatch until you feel the need to breathe in again. Breathe in through your nose without gulping air. The number of seconds you counted before breathing in gives you your control pause.

The ideal control pause is 60 seconds, but a control pause of 40 to 60 denotes good health. A control pause of 30 means you are breathing enough for two people and you are mildly asthmatic. A control pause of 15 indicates that you are breathing for *four* people: this is serious hyperventilation, with asthma symptoms which are likely to occur every day. A control pause of 10 denotes severe asthma with daily and nightly symptoms, medication every day, steroids and hospitalisation from time to time, while a control pause of less than five in a person with asthma means you are having an asthma attack – or calling an ambulance!

prednisone and becotide). It is remarkable how little most people know about their medication and there is often a great deal of confusion to sort out about the function of the different drugs and when they should be taken. We advise patients to take 'relievers' only when they need relief, but to take steroids on a regular basis (for more information about orthodox medication, see Chapter Six).

Having covered this important groundwork, the practitioner can now move on to explaining the Buteyko breathing method, which involves a range of exercises to reduce levels of breathing. When the practitioner is sure that everyone understands the basics, the patients practise controlling their breathing for 15–20 minutes.

The exercises can feel strange and difficult to perform, and so the practitioner spends time with each individual, helping everyone in the group to get them right. This skilled personal assessment is crucial to learning the Buteyko method properly, as people may make many individual mistakes as they learn. If these mistakes are not expertly corrected, your breathing may increase even more – making asthma worse.

At this stage, people in the workshop are clearly very interested but still need answers to many questions about such issues as the effects on asthma of the weather, allergies, sport and so on. After answering questions, the practitioner gives 'homework' – specific exercises geared to the individual needs of each member of the group – as well as these reminders:

- to be aware of your breathing.
- to use the Buteyko method as 'natural salbutamol' in case of any asthma problems, only using your puffer if a few minutes of Buteyko breathing doesn't help.
- to breathe through your nose at all times, using tape to keep the mouth closed at night.
- to sleep on your left side with your mouth closed (or for children, on your tummy).
- to stop playing sport for a few days until your asthma improves (see Chapter Seven).
- to break up your sleep and practise Buteyko breathing if you experience asthma attacks at night (see Chapter Eight).

- to keep taking steroids and to use a puffer rather than a nebuliser (see Chapter Six).

This first session usually lasts for about two hours.

Workshop: day two

At the beginning of the second day's workshop, the practitioner asks how many of the group successfully used the Buteyko method to prevent or relieve asthma symptoms. Around half the group usually report an improvement: some managed to head off an asthma attack without using their puffers, while others had fewer problems than usual and (having taped their mouths for the night to prevent hyperventilation) enjoyed a good night's sleep for a change!

More than half of the group will usually report that they used less of their 'reliever' drugs.

Then the practitioner recaps on the lessons of the day before, going through the control pause and the Buteyko breathing again to make sure that people are doing these correctly. At this stage, some people are likely to say that they can't keep their mouths closed all the time because their noses are blocked – often through sinusitis or rhinitis. They are asked to wait: the solution will shortly be revealed!

The practitioner introduces a Buteyko breathing exercise which can open the airways as effectively as a few puffs of salbutamol. After this exercise, the group finds that wheezing, coughing and tightness in the chest disappears, while the nose is not blocked up. Another interesting effect is noticeable too: the group finds that their pulses are going down. This exercise can stop palpitations within a minute and reduce heart beats from 120 to 80 per minute. The practitioner explains who can do this exercise, when and for how long, because there are some people who should not do it at all.

Youngsters in the group are taught special 'children's exercises' which they do with great enthusiasm and enjoyment. Some need to be pushed a little; others need to be slowed down in order to get the greatest benefit from the exercises they are doing.

On this day – as on the next two days – the group

BUTEYKO ESSENTIALS

- According to the Buteyko method, asthma is your body's defence mechanism against overbreathing, or **hyperventilation**.
- Modern medicine treats the symptoms of asthma: the Buteyko method treats the cause – which is hyperventilation.
- It doesn't matter how many times you breathe each minute: what matters is **how much** air you use each minute.
- The way to cure asthma is to normalise your breathing pattern. This means that your control pause (see page 75) should ideally be 60 when you are at rest.
- To learn the Buteyko method you need to be under the care of a qualified practitioner for a few days.
- You can have a hyperventilation problem without developing asthma, but you will have other health problems. The Buteyko method is also effective for controlling some 150 of the world's commonest diseases, which are the diseases from which 90 per cent of people suffer.

---

practise the Buteyko breathing method a great deal. Again, 'homework' is given, tailored to their needs as adults or children and depending on whether their asthma is mild or severe. Some members of the group may be advised to do physical exercise or to play sport – but without using their puffers beforehand.

Workshop: day three

By day three, everyone in the group is feeling much better than they were when they started learning the Buteyko method. Many of them have reduced their need for 'reliever' medicines by 80 to 100 per cent. All who have been taping their mouths at night are sleeping better. Many of them (especially those who are overweight) report a reduction or loss of appetite, a consequence of their newly improved metabolic processes.

The practitioner discusses the Buteyko approach to diet (see Chapter Ten) and explains the basic rule that you should only eat when you feel hungry. He or she gives a brief outline of the foods which are considered 'good' and 'bad' from a Buteyko point of view, but avoids spending too much time on this discussion, stressing that breathing is more important than diet.

Again, as on previous days, everyone in the group practises the Buteyko method. It is noticeable that children make much faster progress than adults, having spent fewer years being damaged by medication and hyperventilation.

Some patients are keen to stop taking their steroid drugs, but the practitioner works hard to persuade them that they should persevere with steroids – at least until they discuss the matter with their doctor.

FRESH AIR

Is it good to have all the windows in your house closed in order to have more carbon dioxide? Is it good to be on an overloaded bus where many people are exhaling carbon dioxide? It is not, because:

- Neither of these situations will enable you to increase your level of carbon dioxide. Even if there were ten of you in a telephone booth, the level of carbon dioxide would go up to 0.5 per cent, yet if you are asthmatic, you need to raise your level by 2–3 per cent.
- We need fresh air not because of oxygen (the air around us contains 20 per cent oxygen, even on a crowded bus) but because of negative ions. Air conditioners, which also reduce negative ions, are bad for breathing too.
- People on the crowded bus produce not only carbon dioxide but other gases which are detrimental to breathing.

Spirits in the group are generally high, as people say they have made it through the day without using reliever drugs for the first time for maybe 15 or 20 years. Others have been able to play sports – again for the first time – without using their puffers before and after the exercise.

The practitioner gives out more individually tailored 'homework'. Patients are reminded to visit their doctor after the course to discuss modification of their steroid doses.

Workshop: day four

Today, everyone in the group is feeling much better (except perhaps those with emphysema, who are merely feeling better; they will need a little more time before they also feel *much* better).

Most people have stopped using their 'reliever' medicines, while others have cut their usage by around 90 per cent. Some overweight people have lost a kilo or more (2–3 lb) – without making an effort to do so. Everyone's control pause is longer, and hyperventilation has greatly decreased all round. Pulse rates in the group are also down to normal, while people are breathing through their noses without experiencing problems of getting blocked.

Again, we practise the Buteyko breathing exercises, while children may be given some exercises specially designed for their needs, and again the group goes home with individual 'homework' tasks to perform.

Workshop: day five

Having checked control pauses and practised the Buteyko exercises, it is time for our farewell talk. There are many questions still to answer, such as what other diseases the Buteyko method treats. (The answer is an enormous number, including high blood pressure, chronic fatigue, epilepsy and cystic fibrosis).

Everybody is given a strategy to keep normalising their breathing, plus advice about what to do about any future problems. The 'end of workshop' questionnaire is filled in with many positive comments about being able to give up reliever drugs without fear of asthma – often for the first time in decades.

There are questions too about Professor Buteyko, his life and current circumstances (answered in Chapter One of this book). The group generally wants to talk more

about why the Buteyko method is not more widely practised – and why it is still not accepted by the medical
profession and asthma 'experts'. Nearly all of them want
to join a Buteyko support group and to have more information about Buteyko – such as this book.

Emotion is high on this last day because the group is so
pleased and relieved to have found a way to prevent
asthma without drugs. There is much shaking of hands,
and sometimes even applause for the practitioner.

People who have completed a Buteyko workshop say
that these five days have brought more improvement in
their asthma than a lifetime of medication. This is the
Buteyko method.

TYPES OF BREATHING

- It is a common mistake to divide breathing into
  'diaphragmatic', 'chest' and 'stomach' breathing – as
  physiotherapists tend to do.
- We all breathe diaphragmatically because the diaphragm
  is the main breathing muscle which follows 'commands'
  from our breathing centre.
- 'Breathing from the diaphragm' is not going to make you
  healthier – unless you are advised to breathe less, not
  more.
- There are only two types of breathing: normal and
  abnormal. The latter leads to disease.

CHAPTER SIX

Getting the Best out of Drug Treatments

'I firmly believe that if the whole materia medica, as now used, could be sunk to the bottom of the sea, it would be all the better for mankind – and all the worse for the fishes.'

Oliver Wendell Holmes MD, 1860.

If you are one of the three million asthmatics in the UK today who is prescribed drugs for asthma, like it or not you are part of a huge and complex system of doctors, hospitals, health service providers and drugs manufacturers. This system has many political and economic facets – from the growth of drug companies to the increase in the numbers of asthma institutes – and it is expanding every year.

Yet all drugs – and especially the drugs which many asthmatics take every day – create adverse reactions, some of them severe. In America, eminent doctors have argued that billions of wasted dollars, hundreds of thousands of unnecessary hospitalisations for the harmful side effects of drugs – as well as thousands of unnecessary deaths – are the price which society now pays for the promotional excesses of the drug industry.

The situation in the UK is very similar. Here, the cost of NHS asthma treatments has reached £750 million a year. Until the present century, asthma was not even considered to be a potentially fatal illness, yet today, approximately 2,000 people a year in the UK die from asthma. Up to a third of these are of people who did not consider themselves to have severe asthma. Meanwhile, the disease is still on the increase and the death rate from asthma has not decreased for 40 years.

So let's have a look at the contrast between orthodox treatment and the Buteyko method over the years, and then see what the current asthma drugs can do for you – and how you can feel better with **less** of them, not more.

The history of asthma and modern medicine

- 15th–17th centuries: Asthma regarded as a 'slight ailment which promotes longevity'. Remedies of the time include horse riding and syrup of garlic.
- 19th century: Henry Salter, the prominent Victorian physician, writes that 'asthma never kills'. Remedies include tobacco smoking, coffee, gold, morphine and cold baths.
- 1900–1920: Asthma still not regarded as a fatal disease in many medical schools and institutes.
- 1930s: Adrenaline (a bronchodilator) widely used as a drug treatment for asthma. First deaths from this disease are reported.
- 1940s: Isoprenaline (another bronchodilator) is introduced. Deaths from asthma increase.
- 1948: There is a suggestion that use of adrenaline spray

treatment has resulted in a five-fold increase in asthma mortality.

- 1950–1965: Deaths from aminophyllin occur in hospitals in the UK and US.
- 1960s: High-dose isoprenaline is introduced, to be taken through nebulisers. Asthma deaths in New Zealand, Australia and the UK follow.
- 1970s: Sale of bronchodilators decreases. Death rate from asthma also decreases.
- 1976: Fenoteral (a long-lasting bronchodilator) introduced in New Zealand. Seven thousand people per year die, over a five-year period.
- 1982: Scientists recognise that home nebulisers can be dangerous, at times fatal.
- 1989: Studies report that inhaled fenoteral is associated with asthma deaths in New Zealand.
- 1993: Cases of sudden respiratory arrest reported in otherwise healthy young asthmatics treated with salmeterol.
- 1994: Inhaled steroids are associated with psychiatric and endocrine disorders.
- 1996: High-dose bronchodilators suspected of interfering with anti-inflammatory and anti-asthma effects of inhaled steroids.
    - Concerns raised regarding the safety of salmeterol.
    - Evidence that regular use of bronchodilators – even as little as two puffs (200 mcg) – a day may contribute to worsening asthma.
    - Inhaled steroids implicated in glaucoma.

(Details of relevant research papers can be found in the References section on page 183.)

WHY DIDN'T PEOPLE DIE OF ASTHMA
100 YEARS AGO?

There is a great deal of evidence that asthma was not even considered a potentially fatal illness until this century. On the contrary, early medical books express the view that people with asthma – although sometimes suffering terribly from this disease – actually lived longer than people without asthma!

Before 1920, many leading authorities believed that death from asthma was rare, although deaths from other lung diseases (such as emphysema and obstructive pulmonary disease) were sometimes wrongly attributed to asthma – which, in its original definition, simply meant 'hard to breathe'. Asthma mortality rates in young people were stable for a century before the 'epidemic' of asthma deaths in the 1960s.

Since then, despite the advances which medical science claims it has made in understanding the underlying pathophysiological mechanisms of asthma, and in spite of 'advances' in drug treatments, deaths from asthma in young patients have not declined, and in some areas of the world they have increased.

Asthma mortality rates began to increase with the commercial development of powerful bronchodilators such as adrenaline and ephedrine, and reached a peak in the 1960s with the use and overuse of even more powerful bronchodilators and nebulisers (an electric pump which delivers a much bigger dose of a bronchodilating drug).

According to the Italian Professor V. Serafini, 'at this time [1992] when mortality from other chronic diseases is on the decline, clinical observations in recent years have demonstrated an increase in the mortality from asthma in several countries.'

Why should this be? According to Professor Buteyko, asthmatics die from deep breathing which has been made worse by two things:

- Overdose of bronchodilators.
- Lack of steroids.

He notes that people began to die from asthma **after** the development of powerful bronchodilator drugs, because in overdose these 'break' the body's own defence mechanisms. Home nebulisers are suspected on having led to an epidemic of asthma deaths in New Zealand, England and Australia.

In more recent years, the overuse of bronchodilators has been followed by the overuse of steroid drugs – which can also be fatal in the long run. Overdosing on steroids does not kill you immediately, but it may suppress or even destroy the production of natural steroids by your adrenal glands.

Then, because you are reluctant to take yet more steroids (perhaps because of their side effects, or because of the current prejudice against them), you may develop steroid deficiency. This in turn can lead to a severe asthma attack, hospitalisation and even death.

Surveys have shown that up to 30 per cent of people who die from asthma did not consider themselves to be severely asthmatic. It could well be that they are young people irritated by their lack of breath during sport or sex, or when they have a cold or the flu. So they took one puff of their bronchodilator after another, and then another and another... eventually with tragic consequences.

The history of asthma and the Buteyko method

Research between 1971 and 1996 establishes that:

- Hyperventilation and low carbon dioxide (hypocapnia) are common in asthma.
- Low levels of carbon dioxide are the rule in asthma (until respiratory failure sets in).
- Carbon dioxide is a bronchodilator and protects against bronchospasm.
- Asthma improves with breathing control.
- Tests using peak flow meters are known to cause bronchospasm, making test results unreliable, especially for people with a long history of asthma.
- Breathing retraining for people with asthma leads to profound improvements in general health and in asthma in particular.

Bronchodilators

It is some 70 years since physicians started to prescribe the powerful bronchodilator drugs adrenaline and ephedrine to 'open the airways' of people with asthma. In that time, different and even more powerful bronchodilators have been developed, and today salbutamol has emerged as the UK's most frequently prescribed bronchodilator drug.

Bronchodilators are also known as 'relievers' because they 'rescue' you from the unpleasant symptoms of asthma – as opposed to 'preventers', the steroid medicines which prevent asthma symptoms. None of these drugs can cure asthma; they can only provide temporary relief from the symptoms.

The best way to 'keep asthma under control' – as most doctors aim to do – is to use a bronchodilator (or salbutamol 'puffer') for emergencies, and to use steroids for prevention of emergencies. It is important that bronchodilators should be used not according to a rigid timetable, but only when you feel that you need it, in the same way as you would take a headache tablet for a headache. In other words, if you don't have any asthma symptoms, don't use this drug.

People often give the following reasons for taking bronchodilators:

- I have a low peak flow.
- I need to open up my airways before taking a preventer such as becotide.
- I want to play sports.
- I always take it.
- My doctor recommended it.

But these are **not** good reasons for taking bronchodilators.

Nor is salbutamol any use for a wheeze or cough. It is intended to relieve bronchospasm, not coughing.

Some people who have been taking it for years ask me whether they should cut their dosage in half – or even give it up altogether. My answer is – just don't take bronchodilators when you don't need them, that's all. Take them when you need them, and take one puff only each time. Why take two puffs as a matter of routine when it may be absolutely unnecessary to take a double dose?

Short-term relief, long-term trouble

It is important to avoid taking bronchodilator drugs unnecessarily for some very good reasons.

- Firstly, they don't cure asthma, because they don't address the cause of asthma.
- Secondly, they can cause nausea, vomiting, loss of appetite, abdominal discomfort, hyperactivity (especially in children), personality changes, rapid pulse, heart irregularity, dizziness, anxiety, delirium, hallucinations and more.
- Thirdly, and most importantly, they cause further hyperventilation.
- Finally, an overdose of bronchodilators can be fatal. Approximately 2,000 patients now die from asthma every year, and fears have grown in recent years that inappropriate use of bronchodilator drugs have contributed to the rise in the death rate. In the 1960s after the introduction of a new, high-dose over-the-counter bronchodilator (isoprenaline), a virtual epidemic of asthma deaths hit Britain. After a good deal of adverse publicity following the death of Brian Jones of the Rolling Stones, this drug was withdrawn.

Deaths from asthma had increased eightfold between 1959 and 1966. According to the *British Medical Journal* in 1968:

Since increasing proportions of the deaths have been certified by coroners, sudden and unexpected deaths appear to be becoming more frequent, and we must suspect that modern treatment which is so helpful to most patients, may be a serious hazard to a few. The period of rising mortality coincides with increasing use of both corticosteroid drugs and pressurized broncho-dilator aerosols, especially of isoprenaline.

In the 1980s a series of deaths occurred in New Zealand after the introduction of another high-dose bronchodila-tor. Again, the drug was withdrawn – and the number of deaths dropped. Some years later a study from Canada found that asthma patients using twice the recommended daily dose of bronchodilators had double the risk of a fatal or near-fatal asthma attack. This is thought to be because these drugs can cause increased sensitivity to allergens in what is called the 'rebound' effect, as well as long-term deterioration of lung function.

But perhaps the most relevant – but little known – reason for avoiding unnecessary doses of bronchodilators is that although they provide short-term relief, in the long term they make asthma worse. This is because by open-ing up your airways they make you hyperventilate even more than before, worsening your breathing pattern and causing you more severe problems with asthma in the future.

Long-term relievers – serious trouble?

There are worries too about the safety and effectiveness of the new class of bronchodilator, salmeterol. This drug is a long-acting, slow-release bronchodilator which can be taken once every 12 hours and is prescribed only for use on a regular basis, two puffs at a time.

You are supposed to use this drug in the morning and before bed at night, without even knowing whether you are going to need it. Yet this is a powerful drug, at least ten times stronger than salbutamol. Surely it is unwise to use it blindly in this way?

Some asthmatics say to me, 'But when I use salmeterol I don't need to use salbutamol because I don't have any asthma symptoms!' I say, 'Well, if you used morphine for a headache you'd find that it works better than other headache tablets. But there is a problem. Morphine will destroy you – especially if you take it twice a day every day! And what can help you after morphine? Not an ordinary headache tablet for sure.'

Emergency action

So what **should** you do if you are a severe asthmatic and you are having an asthma attack which is so serious that one, two or even three puffs of salbutamol don't help? In such a case you **must** take oral steroids to prevent further more serious symptoms, because this is a sign that an even more severe asthma attack is coming on.

IN A NUTSHELL

- Use bronchodilators strictly on a 'when required' basis.
- Use the minimum dose to get relief from symptoms.
- Don't use long-lasting bronchodilators.
- If two to three puffs of salbutamol don't help you, then take oral steroids.

A CURE FOR ASTHMA?

From the beginnings of recorded history, people have tried to combat the symptoms of asthma with all sorts of weird and wonderful potions. Some of the first ever 'asthma medicines' contain chemical compounds which have been reproduced in modern drugs: others seem totally grotesque and bizarre to us today. But what will history's verdict be on the massive doses of bronchodilators and steroids handed out with full confidence by 20th-century doctors? Will they seem any less strange? Time will tell.

- Four thousand years ago, the Chinese doctor Ma Huan was making medicines for asthma from the herb ephedra. The asthma drug ephedrine – derived from the same plant – was rediscovered in Japan in 1914 and is still in use.
- The influential physician Galen, born in Asia Minor in AD 131, recommended owls' blood in wine as the best remedy for asthma.
- Sir John Floyer, the prominent British physician, included a list of asthma remedies in his *Treatise of the Asthma* (1698), such as 'Gill and Hyslop', 'Syrop of Sulphur' and 'Spirit of Hartshorn' – as well as bleeding and purging. His treatise was translated into French and German and had a great influence on English clinicians of the 18th century.
- Other 18th-century remedies for asthma included 'Syrop of Garlick', 'Tincture of Lavender', 'Smoked Amber with Tobacco' and 'Gentle Vomiting'.
- By the 19th century, people with asthma were being dosed with a wide range of potions from chloroform and belladonna to strong coffee, tobacco and alcohol.
- In 1863 the leading physician Henry Salter wrote about

'the treatment of the asthmatic paroxysm by full doses of alcohol'. He described the case of an asthmatic woman who seemed to be beyond all help. He had tried everything – chloroform, ipecacuanha, strong coffee, iodide of potassium, tobacco smoked in a pipe, cigars – but nothing worked. Only when she was recommended to try gin did she apparently gain instant relief from her symptoms!

- In 1834 the *Edinburgh Medical Journal* came close to understanding what we now know to be 'triggers' for asthma when they gave 'scientific' reasons why people with asthma should not use feather pillows. The journal reported an 'urgent case of asthma (which) appeared to be induced by electricity excited by new feathers'.

- Victorian doctors used blood-letting, cold baths, mineral water, electricity and magnetism to treat asthma – all in vain.

- Chloroform became a very fashionable remedy after Queen Victoria inhaled it during the birth of Prince Leopold. Indeed 'Anaesthesia' was a popular girls' Christian name for years to come. But in 1833 an encyclopedia of practical medicine had warned doctors that chloroform was a 'remedy not free from risk'. It wasn't until 1928, however, that the august *British Medical Journal* confirmed that view by reporting a few deaths of asthmatics from using chloroform.

- Towards the end of the 19th century, a Dr Oliver discovered adrenaline. Sir Henry Dale purified the chemical messenger it contains, and adrenaline – together with ephedrine – were used as powerful bronchodilators from the 1920s onward.

- In North America, a number of folk remedies were available for asthma, as reported in *Magical Medicine* (1907) by W. Hand:

    – Nebraskans kept cats to 'catch' their asthma.

    – Texans blew into the mouths of frogs before daylight believing that the frog would die of their asthma, leaving them cured.

    – New Yorkers nailed a lock of the asthmatic's hair to a tree in the hope that the tree would die but that the asthmatic would be well.

    – Nova Scotians stood in the hot blood of a slaughtered animal to cure asthma.

    – The early inhabitants of Los Angeles thought that owning a Chihuahua dog was the solution.

    – In Kentucky and in Oregon people measured their children against the wall in the hope – familiar to modern parents and doctors – that when children grew, they would 'outgrow' their asthma.

- In 1997, thousands of Indian people lined up for a folk cure for asthma which involved swallowing a live goldfish – which would in turn 'swallow' the asthma as it went down.

Yet through all these centuries and with all these misconceived ideas, people did not die of asthma...

Steroids

The group of drugs known as steroids (or corticosteroids) was developed earlier this century from the hormone cortisol, which is naturally produced in our bodies by the outer layer of the adrenal gland. The first steroid drug, cortisone, was in fact a natural hormone and modern corticosteroid drugs are all chemically similar to the natural hormones.

Interest in steroids intensified during the 1940s when researchers found that they could have dramatic results in the treatment of rheumatoid arthritis, and the scientists who had isolated and purified cortisone were awarded the Nobel Prize for Medicine in 1950.

Soon cortisone was being tried for a wide variety of medical conditions – with some striking successes. One of these conditions was asthma. It very quickly became clear that steroids could combat severe, life-threatening attacks of asthma. However, disappointing relapses occurred when steroids were withdrawn and before long it emerged that long-term maintenance treatment was essential in some patients.

But like most powerful drugs, steroids proved to have some major side effects. Most seriously, they suppress the immune system, making the patient more vulnerable to a host of other diseases. As a result, in the late 1960s there was a reaction against the use of steroids. Nevertheless, these drugs have saved hundreds of thousands of asthmatics' lives. One intravenous injection of steroids in hospital during a severe asthma attacks makes it possible for you to breathe again – and to survive.

Some people with severe asthma who have suffered side

effects from steroids in the past now refuse to take these drugs. Yet it is an **overdose** of steroids which produces side effects. Surviving on the razor edge of severe asthma, it is only a matter of time before such as person is admitted to hospital where – in order to save their life – they will be given a massive dose of steroids, which in turn will suppress and damage the production of their own natural steroids by their adrenal glands. If asthmatics then – through fear of side effects – neglect to take more steroids, they may develop steroid deficiency. This in turn may lead to such a severe asthmatic attack that even nebulisers don't help – and so it's back to hospital again. Sometimes, too late.

In this vicious circle of steroid depletion, hyperventilation is also damaging to the adrenal glands which produce the body's natural steroids. Some asthmatics develop steroid deficiency as a result of serious or prolonged hyperventilation. If they do, they must take artificial steroids or put their lives at risk, just as diabetics must inject insulin when their own natural insulin fails.

According to Professor Buteyko, oral steroids are in fact the best medication for asthma because steroids are the only drugs which can reduce hyperventilation, addressing the cause of asthma – in contrast to bronchodilators which increase it.

Professor Buteyko believes that asthmatics die not from asthma but from hyperventilation caused by two factors:

- Overdose of bronchodilators.
- Lack of steroids.

SIDE EFFECTS OF STEROIDS

Steroids used in an inhaler have few significant side effects as the dose is very small. However, you may experience:

- hoarseness (the most common complaint)
- candida or 'thrush' (a yeast-like fungus in the mouth)
- suppression of growth for some children

Inhaled steroids are now also implicated in the development of psychiatric and endocrine disorders.

Oral steroids can have more serious side effects, including:

- suppression of the body's production of natural steroids
- reactivation of latent infections (such as tuberculosis)
- the breakdown of partly healed stomach or adrenal ulcers
- excessive hairiness (hirsutism)
- a moon-like face
- excessive appetite and weight gain

In addition, if you already have diabetes, osteoporosis, glaucoma or cataracts, steroids can make these worse.

But note: most of these side effect occur as a result of **improper use** of steroids. Taking steroids twice a day every day for months on end – whether the drugs are needed or not – as many doctors recommend, is the real cause of unpleasant side effects, especially the suppression of your own natural steroids.

How steroids work

The medical profession admits to understanding little about how steroids work. Unfortunately this lack of understanding has serious implications for the drug treatment of people with asthma because steroids are often given in **overdose** (too large a quantity) or in **underdose** (too little).

Fortunately, Professor Buteyko discovered how steroids work. He realised that these drugs decrease breathing, which treats any inflammation, reduces mucus and helps to relieve bronchospasm.

Steroids are also known to protect against allergy. From the Buteyko point of view this is because reduction in breathing creates more carbon dioxide in the body – which in turn makes the immune system strong, so protecting against allergy.

How to make the most of steroids

The right way to take steroids, according to the Buteyko method, is in response to your condition. As all asthmatics know, that can vary a great deal from day to day. Every person with asthma should have a clear understanding of what steroids do, how to take them and when.

No doctor can monitor your condition on a day-to-day basis, which means it is up to you to assess your own condition and administer the correct dose, according to your condition, your breathing, your control pause and your pulse. But when your body needs steroids, give it steroids. You need to learn about your own asthma, and to understand the signs which tell you that your body needs steroids – oral or inhaled – now!

This is preferable to developing a 'steroid debt' which your body will not forget or forgive. Pay the debt sooner rather than later; if you don't, other people in hospital soon will – and with a massively bigger dose than the one you have been avoiding.

The ideal treatment for asthma is to practise the Buteyko method of breathing control and meanwhile to use steroids when necessary. Ultimately, the Buteyko method will reduce overbreathing – and so inflammation and allergy will also be reduced – while increasing your natural production of steroids. In time, there will be no need to use the artificial ones any longer.

The **wrong** way to take steroids is according to a doctor's schedule or 'five-day plan', in which you are told in advance how many steroids to take and when. How does your doctor know what dose you are going to need in three days' time or more? The same goes for inhaled steroids. Some days you will need more than two puffs twice a day; on other days you will need less.

And why are you being told to take these 'preventer' drugs in the morning, when the night – which is the most difficult and dangerous time for asthmatics – has already passed? The best time to take steroids is two or three hours before bedtime to prevent early morning problems. (If you have an asthma attack in the morning however and find that two or three puffs of Ventolin don't help, take steroids straight away to prevent more serious problems.)

The best way to take oral steroids is to chew up the tablet and wash it down with a drink of warm water (not milk, which is bad for asthma). This helps you to absorb the tablets better with a minimum of irritation to the stomach. You'll feel the effects sooner, too – after two or three hours instead of six or eight. It is usually recommended that you take steroids after food, but I have found it is better to take them on an empty stomach.

If you are on a 'scheme' which is supposed to reduce your dose of steroids but you feel that your asthma is getting worse, **don't reduce your dose**. Increase it instead and return to that level of dosage when you feel better.

Many people with asthma believe they are 'hooked' on steroids and will have to take them for the rest of their lives. This is not true. The good news is that by practising the Buteyko method so that you achieve a control pause of 40, even people who have been taking big doses of oral steroids are able to get off the steroid hook.

Cromoglycate drugs

When the first commercial cromoglycate drug appeared in the 1960s it was hailed as a revolution in asthma treatment: 'Asthma cure discovered!' proclaimed the

---

IN A NUTSHELL

To make the best use of steroids:

- Estimate your condition and establish the correct dosage for you.
- Change the dosage daily depending on how you improve or deteriorate.
- Explain this plan to your doctor, who should help you to follow it.

---

newspaper headlines. Alas, nothing so remarkable has happened and the great revolution has failed.

The drug concerned was cromoglycate, which doctors believe has little if any effect on adults, but which is commonly prescribed for children with asthma. Doctors argue that cromoglycate has few significant side effects and often recommend it as a preferred line of treatment before steroids.

Yet very little is known about how this drug works, and according to Professor Buteyko, it does have significant side effects. He found that it makes the bronchotubes inflexible, comparable to the lung damage suffered by people who have worked in the mining or cement industries. He also found that these drugs may cause bronchitis after just a few weeks of regular use.

To sum up, these drugs don't stop asthma attacks and they don't reduce breathing (as steroids do). **Don't use them**.

Methylxanthines

This group of drugs – which includes the asthma medications theophylline and aminophylline – can also open up your airways. Theophylline, like caffeine, stimulates your central nervous system. How these drugs work is not fully understood, but it is known that theophylline relaxes bronchial muscles when given in the correct dosage.

Unfortunately, too much theophylline can cause convulsions and – ultimately – death. Children and old people are most vulnerable to the severe side effects of an overdose of theophylline because of the complexity of selecting

ALISON, AGED 50

I've gone from thinking my life will always be governed by asthma and drugs to feeling totally in control of what's happening. This is the best thing I've ever 'bought' in my life.

the correct dose. When used in conjunction with inhaled bronchodilators – as some doctors recommend – these drugs can be fatal.

Under the circumstances, the most important thing I can say about these drugs is **don't use them.**

Peak flow meters

A peak flow meter is a device used – either at home or in your GP's surgery – to measure the volume of your 'forced expiration'. In other words, you blow into it as hard as you can to produce a reading which tells you your ability to blow out air. A lot of air is considered 'good'.

But not only can peak flow meters be harmful to people with asthma; their results are also unreliable and misleading, telling you nothing about your breathing patterns or about hyperventilation. They can also set up a vicious circle of needing more bronchodilators to maintain a good peak flow, therefore increasing hyperventilation and – in turn – asthma symptoms. One study (Gayrard et al, see References page 184) described peak flow as 'a crude measure of broncoconstriction' which 'cannot alone provide conclusive evidence of asthma'.

Many people with asthma develop wheezing, coughing and/or tightness in the chest after using a peak flow meter. This is because when you blow into the device, you blow out a lot of carbon dioxide – which switches on your body's defence mechanism of bronchoconstriction.

Many people have great peak flow figures – when they feel well or when they have just used a nebuliser – but may be struck by an asthma attack within hours. In fact, the bigger your lung capacity, the bigger your potential hyperventilation – and so the worse your asthma attack may be. Developing a good lung capacity can certainly help you in sport or running or carrying a piano up to the sixth floor – but it's better to get rid of your asthma first. (It's worth noting too that some non-asthmatics have a small peak flow.)

Doctors underline the necessity to maintain 'good' peak flow figures, but if you enter this never-ending battle you are bound to lose. Say your peak flow reading is 400 (which is considered pretty good for asthmatics). To maintain this figure, you take asthma drugs such as bronchodilators – which increase your hyperventilation, making your asthma symptoms worse in the long run. The logic of this situation is that you have to keep increasing your dose of asthma drugs – which means increasing your asthma problem – in order to keep up your peak flow readings.

Clearly, a no-win scenario.

Alternatively, you can measure your asthma by checking your control pause (see page 75). This is far more relevant to your problem – and safer too.

Physiotherapy

Many people who end up in hospital after an asthma

attack are offered physiotherapy as a form of treatment for their symptoms. Alternatively, some doctors will refer their asthmatic patients to physiotherapists for treatment in the surgery. Although there has been very little research to demonstrate the effectiveness of physiotherapy in the treatment of asthma, it has been used for decades.

Unfortunately, physiotherapy for asthma involves teaching you to breathe more deeply – in the belief that you need more oxygen. It also involves 'coughing' therapy, in which the physiotherapist teaches you how to cough in order to remove mucus from your lungs.

However, not only do both these techniques increase hyperventilation, making asthma worse, but, by removing mucus, physiotherapy is also working against one of your body's defence mechanisms against loss of carbon dioxide.

In Australia, at the time of writing, around a dozen physiotherapists have stopped treating asthmatics with these techniques and have instead turned to the Buteyko method (see case study on page 17).

My advice on physiotherapy for asthma: **don't use it.**

Complementary treatments

This book is not the place to discuss these treatments in detail, but from a Buteyko point of view the main principle to consider is – what effect do complementary therapies have on breathing?

Any therapy which increases breathing, such as physiotherapy, rebirthing (which involves deep breathing), blowing up balloons – as practised in some hospitals – is harmful. All breathing exercises, which should be called deep breathing exercises, are harmful. If you have asthma, you don't need any practice at deep breathing; you've already been doing it for years!

Any therapy which decreases breathing even indirectly and temporarily, such as relaxation, meditation, the Alexander technique, acupuncture, massage, a vegetarian diet (because eating protein increases hyperventilation), fasting (because eating increases hyperventilation), Tai Chi (which is relaxing) – will do good rather than bad.

Yoga is a wonderful way to control body, mind and spirit and can therefore be very beneficial for people with asthma. Most yoga positions and exercises help you to retain carbon dioxide because the positions you are required to hold, reduce breathing. Unfortunately, most western yoga teachers recommend deep or 'full' breathing, which they believe will help you 'get more oxygen'.

A true yogi, by contrast, should be able to control breathing, with the capacity to breathe very deeply, very shallowly or hardly at all. But these are exercises for special effects. What counts is the breathing of a yogi when he is not doing these yoga exercises. What is his breathing pattern? It should be very shallow and superficial.

Wonderful as yoga can be, there is one problem: as a therapy it is too empirical. In other words, you don't know where you are going or what is going on with your breathing. Like other forms of relaxation and meditation, it is good to lower your breathing for an hour or more each day – but you breathe for 24 hours a day. What really counts is what is happening to your breathing during the other 23.

Some therapies, such as Traditional Chinese Medicine, homeopathy and yoga can be good **or** bad – depending upon the practitioner. Sport can be good or bad – depending on whether you have learned to control your breathing using Buteyko techniques.

Other self-help methods of reducing asthma are simple and effective common sense, such as:

- Get rid of any chronic infection you may have.
- Get rid of carpets which attract dust and other allergens.
- Breathe through your nose.
- Avoid stress.
- Eat healthy food, not mass-produced junk.

Going to hospital

What happens when you arrive in hospital with a severe asthma attack? Naturally, you expect the best available treatment and care. But whether or not you will get it is another matter. Let's run through the typical treatment in a typical UK hospital.

The first step in the management of your acute condition will probably be to give you a bronchodilator drug, administered either by a nebuliser or by injection. If you show any signs of oxygen deficiency or an unusually fast pulse you will most likely be given oxygen through a mask. Almost everyone admitted to hospital with an asthma attack is given oxygen in this way.

But few doctors understand why you have an oxygen shortfall in the first place. During a severe asthma attack you are suffering from a lack of oxygen because you are hyperventilating acutely. Artificial administration of oxygen makes you feel even worse, so that your condition gets worse, not better, and you may develop bronchospasm.

More dangerous still is the fact that oxygen therapy can cause pulmonary collapse and respiratory failure. This is because when high concentrations of oxygen are breathed for many hours, they are toxic to the tiny air sacs (alveoli) and blood vessels (pulmonary capillaries) in the lungs. Another effect of administering pure oxygen is to cause nausea, ringing in the ears and twitching of the face, symptoms which warn of convulsions to come. The fact that pure oxygen is toxic has been known for a hundred years, yet it is still being used . . .

You will **still** not have received a steroid drug – and this delay, I believe, is one of the main causes of death from asthma. Only after all other measures have failed – after about an hour of ineffective, even damaging treatments – are steroids used.

Even if you have been given steroids and your condition has improved, a nurse is likely to come around every hour to put you on a nebuliser – giving you a large dose of bronchodilators to make you hyperventilate again. Then a physiotherapist may be called in to 'help you with coughing'. But this so called 'coughing technique' is yet another way to make you hyperventilate more – again causing loss of oxygen and leading to bronchospasm.

How to survive in hospital

Professor Buteyko advises you insist on the following treatment should you ever be admitted to hospital with an asthma attack:

- Make sure you are given an intravenous steroid drug as soon as possible after they put you on a nebuliser (which is almost unavoidable). You will feel better within a few minutes, after which you will be able to refuse a routine nebuliser treatment.

- Accept treatment with a nebuliser only if you feel you really need it – and for just enough time to get relief from your symptoms.
- Refuse to take oxygen.
- Refuse any physiotherapy which involves blowing up balloons, coughing therapy and other forms of hyper-ventilation.

Of course, it can be very difficult to assert your wishes under the circumstances of an acute asthma attack, so it may be wise to brief your partner or relatives so that they can communicate what you want – as well as keeping an eye on your continuing treatment. (Remember: Dr Semmelweis?)

After hospital

The two weeks after leaving hospital are an anxious time with a high risk of relapsing into acute asthma. Why should this be the case? Again, the misuse and misunder-standing of steroids is the root of the problem.

What usually happens is that after leaving hospital you are advised to take a high daily dose of steroids, say 50 mg, and then to reduce that dose by 5 mg every three days. Or, you may be prescribed what they call a 'steroid burst' for five days only, stopping steroids completely after this time. You may also be given a complicated combination of neb-ulisers and long-acting bronchodilators.

The trouble is, no matter how good your doctor is, he or she cannot know what will happen to you in three days'

DEAR DOCTOR . . .

Sooner rather than later you should discuss the Buteyko approach to asthma with your doctor. The following points – which you could put in the form of a letter – might help you to approach him or her fully armed with the scientific facts. (Should you wish to study the subject further, seek out some of the published papers listed in the References section on page 183.)

- Asthma is a breathing disorder.
- According to scientific international norms I am supposed to breathe between four and six litres of air in one minute while I am at rest. I breathe three times as much as this (as demonstrated by my minute volume).
- I am overbreathing, which means that while I am taking in more oxygen, less oxygen is actually getting to certain areas of my brain and body (Verigo-Bohr effects, see page 48).
- At the same time I am exhaling too much carbon dioxide which is a smooth-muscle relaxant and bronchodilator. This means that my bronchotubes become constricted.
- As a result of this I have been prescribed chemical bronchodilators which have been implicated in recent asthma deaths and rising morbidity.

time after you have been discharged from hospital. Your asthma may get worse – but according to your doctor's plan, you have to decrease your dose of steroids. It could be that on the very day when you are supposed to stop taking steroids altogether, you feel really terrible because you have got flu, or a cold, or your asthma got worse.

Logically, this is a time at which you should be increas-

- Buteyko practitioners claim that Professor Buteyko in 1952 invented a method to change breathing patterns, which could be a drug-free solution to my overbreathing problem.
- The Buteyko method underwent a scientific trial in Australia in 1994–5 showing an unprecedented 90 per cent reduction in the use of bronchodilators, together with a 50 per cent reduction in the use of steroids, by the asthmatics in the trial. The control group, using conventional medicines, showed no reduction in use of bronchodilators or steroids.
- Buteyko practitioners say that when I start learning the Buteyko breathing techniques I must keep taking my steroid medication, but that I should use my 'reliever' (bronchodilator) medicine only when I feel that I need it.
- I plan to learn how to use breathing techniques – in which carbon dioxide acts as a natural salbutamol – to stop the symptoms of asthma. I will keep my puffer in my pocket just in case. I will use it if I need to use it but, I hope, never again.
- Once I have been free from asthma symptoms for a few weeks I will ask you to reduce my dose of steroids.

Your doctor may be sceptical – indeed you may be sceptical to start with – but it quite likely that he or she will say, 'This is just a matter of breathing, so why not try it?'

ing your steroid dose, but your 'plan' tells you to decrease it – or stop it. So what happens next? Hospital again.

This scenario raises several serious questions:

- As we are all different, why are we all prescribed the same 50 mg dose of steroids after hospital?

- Why give us five days to come off steroids – as opposed to three, or seven, or nine – regardless of our condition?

The answer to both these questions is that doctors don't understand how steroids work, they don't know how to detect steroid deficiency or to prescribe the correct dose, and they don't like steroids.

The sad implications of this lack of knowledge about steroids is that they are not used when really needed – resulting in deaths from asthma – and that when they are used, they are often given in overdose, causing the unpleasant symptoms which made people want to avoid them in the first place.

CHAPTER SEVEN

Asthma and Sport

Modern medicine has a variety of explanations for the phenomenon it calls 'exercise-induced asthma'. As far back as the Roman Empire it was recognised that asthma was related to exercise, while the prominent 17th-century British physician Sir John Floyer linked asthma with emotional stress, laughter and exercise. Today, doctors try to explain this link in terms of 'drying out of the airways', which they argue follows the faster, deeper breathing induced by exercise or laughter.

I once attended an asthma conference in Sydney, organised by the Australian Asthma Foundation. The hall was full of health professionals and asthmatics, despite the hefty conference fee. We heard the usual explanations of the virtues of a new drug treatment for asthma, and then someone asked one professor, 'Why do I have asthma during sport?'

The professor said, 'Because your breathing during sport cools down your airways.'

Then another person asked, 'If I were to exercise in a sauna, does that mean I would not develop asthma?'

The professor thought for a minute and then said, 'No, you would develop asthma because the temperature there

HOW TO WALK UPHILL – OR UPSTAIRS – WHEN YOU HAVE ASTHMA

Walking uphill, or even upstairs, can be a real problem for people with severe asthma. Your breathing may become very deep, inducing coughing and wheezing. You are left short of breath and in need of your inhaler.

To avoid these problems, we recommend you follow these simple steps:

- Do not use an inhaler beforehand. Use it when you need it.
- Breathe strictly through your nose as you walk uphill, and breathe as little as possible.
- Walk slowly at first, 'listening' to your own breathing and stopping to rest whenever you feel that you have lost

would still be low enough to cool your airways.' Quite a few people in the hall nearly developed laughter-induced asthma at that reply.

So why *do* people with asthma have problems when they run or laugh, even when the 90°C of a sauna and/or the effects of running in fog or rain are not enough to stop their airways drying out? The Buteyko method solves this age-old problem.

Professor Buteyko points out that if you look at the breathing of somebody who runs, or laughs, or walks upstairs, or plays sport – or who argues, shouts, feels fearful or coughs – you will see that it has one thing in common: hyperventilation. Indeed many children have learned that they can bring on an asthma attack by crying or by these other means – quite useful as a way to manipulate your parents or avoid going to school!

control of your breath.
- Once you have reached the top of the hill – or the stairs – try not to take a deep breath but try to hold back your breathing.

When you can make it to the top in one go without having to stop and rest, then you can try to go faster. As long as you stay in control of your breath, you are safe.

Basically, your ability to walk uphill or upstairs depends upon your control pause. If your CP is less than 5, you will find it hard even to walk across the room. But if it should go as high as 50, you would probably be able to run up to the fifth floor with your mouth closed – and still have no asthma symptoms!

The question remains whether sport benefits people with asthma – or whether it does you harm? There are other related questions too, such as – if sport is good for you, what is the best sport? And what about using your puffer before sport: is this a good idea?

From Buteyko's point of view, sport can be either beneficial **or** harmful – depending on the level of carbon dioxide that you are left with after exercising.

The effect of exercise on your asthma

Let's look at what is going on with your breathing when you take exercise:

- Firstly, your breathing becomes fast and deep. You exhale more carbon dioxide than usual and so your bronchotubes become narrowed.

Moderate and severe asthmatics don't generally have enough carbon dioxide to get past this stage, because their carbon dioxide levels are already so low that any further depletion switches on the body's defence mechanisms in the form of asthma symptoms.

Mild asthmatics may have sufficient reserves of carbon dioxide to go through this stage.

- Secondly, the activity of your muscles speeds up your metabolic processes so that your body starts producing **more** carbon dioxide – which in turn opens up your bronchotubes.

  If you exercise long enough, your level of carbon dioxide may become higher than it was before you started – and so you feel great. This effect may last for a few minutes or several hours, depending on your ability to control your breathing.

- Thirdly, after stopping exercise, your breathing is still deep but your muscles have stopped producing carbon dioxide – and so this is a crucial time for people with asthma. The positive effects of the exercise may stay with you if you can control your breathing, but if you breathe out too much of the carbon dioxide which you accumulated during exercise, you are likely to develop an asthma attack.

To find out how sport affects your asthma, check your carbon dioxide level 15 to 20 minutes after taking exercise. The method is the same as at other times: by measuring your control pause (see page 75).

Say your control pause was 20 before taking exercise

(I wouldn't advocate you play sport if it is any lower because you are likely to have an asthma attack). Things could go one of two ways. Either your control pause will increase to around 23, 25 or even higher. Or, it will go down to around 10 (which means you are wheezing and coughing), or as low as 5 – which means an asthma attack.

Is swimming good for people with asthma?

It is a commonly held view that swimming is an especially good sport for people with asthma, and it's true that there have been Olympic swimming champions who are asthmatics. Many of the Australian swimming team have asthma. They swim for a few hours a day, every day, for years – and yet they still have asthma, and they still take drugs to treat their symptoms.

The optimistic way to look at this is that asthma can't stop you becoming an Olympic champion. On the other hand, pessimists might feel – even though I can become an Olympic champion, I can't stop my asthma!

So is swimming good for you, or not? Apart from the fact that some people develop sensitivity to the chlorine used to sterilise swimming pool water, swimming **can** be good for you. That is, if you can control your breathing so that your carbon dioxide levels stay higher after swimming than they were before you started.

But if that is not the case, you are likely to end up with further asthma symptoms. Indeed, some people with asthma have asthma attacks before they have even left the swimming pool.

How does Buteyko relieve asthma problems?

It is easy to understand why the Buteyko method is good for sport – because almost all sports require either stamina (like running a marathon) or concentration (like shooting or snooker) or thinking (like chess) or all of these things. The exceptions are sports that require short, sharp bursts of energy – it is less important how you breathe during a 100-metre sprint because that is over in about 10 seconds, whereas you might play squash for 40 minutes or more.

• **Stamina** The major problem with all strenuous sports – running, cycling, boxing and so on – is that you get out of breath. This is the first problem that occurs; muscle collapse comes afterwards. Those who can keep going longer in the breathing sense can also do it in the muscular sense – and they are called champions, not only in long-distance running, but in all sorts of sports. The Buteyko method brings more oxygen into the muscles (through breathing less, due to the Bohr effect, see page 48) and teaches you how to control your breathing in a way that no other technique can. The more deeply you breathe the less carbon dioxide you retain, the less oxygen you have in the cells of your muscles, the less stamina you have, the poorer sportsman or woman you are. So that, whenever stamina is involved, the Buteyko method is there to help.

• **Concentration and thinking** Can you imagine a champion on the shooting range hyperventilating, yet still hitting the target? Or a snooker player winning a competition with shaking hands? Shaking hands are a typical problem of hyperventilation, mostly in acute cases (check yourself next time you are going through a family drama, experiencing fear, panic, an asthma attack, anger, etc), but it is there during hidden hyperventilation too. Not in such an obvious form, but enough to make it unlikely that you would achieve much in competitive sport. And even if you are good at a sport, there will be room for improvement, which top sportsmen are always hungry for. It's a bit like a person with one eye playing tennis – however good they are, wouldn't they be better off with two eyes? That's why whether you are an Olympic marksman in Sydney 2000 or a once-a-week darts player after a couple of pints in the pub, you can use the Buteyko method of breath control to do it better.

We all know that sport is good – or even very good – for us. It's self-evident. Isn't it? But if sport is good – or even very good – for your health, why do you develop asthma symptoms from it? (And it is well known that sport triggers asthma attacks – that's why many doctors prescribe as couple of puffs of bronchodilators before sport, as they would before you entered a house full of dust-mites or cats.)

This raises two more questions: why, on the one hand, do you get punished by your asthma for doing a 'good thing' i.e. playing sport? And why, on the other hand, do doctors recommend you to play sport if it brings on asthma problems?

Because traditional medicine can't explain this conundrum, we have to turn to the Buteyko method, to understand that sport itself is not 'bad' (lots of people benefit from it) and not 'good' (lots of people develop a whole range of problems, and not just asthma). Sport is a 'tool' which enables you to perfect your body and health, if you use it properly, or can ruin both if you don't. From a purely physiological point of view, sport is a way of improving the working of many vital organs by increasing oxygen circulation in the blood, eliminating poisonous substances, exercising muscles, heart, lungs, nervous system and – sometimes – the brain as well, **but it is only going to happen if you increase levels of carbon dioxide**.

If, as a result of playing any sport, your level of CO_2 drops – because you exhale more of this gas than your muscle work produces – then you are in trouble: you may develop asthma or even suffer a heart attack – either there and then, on the sports field, or later – because you may be damaging your long-term health. In other words, if your CP before you played sport is higher than it is afterwards, your way of playing sport and your breath control (or rather lack of it) put your body in a corner.

I know many great athletes who have developed serious health problems despite having the 'healthiest' lifestyle one can imagine: no smoking, no drinking, a sensible diet (most of them have their own dietician), lots of vitamins, oxygen and what not – and lots and lots of sport. Few people would realise that these champions' problems arose not despite playing sport but because of it. In 1998 I spoke to a woman who a few years earlier been one of the leading athletes in the UK and she told me that not only had her health deteriorated hugely because of sport but – and I quote – 'All my team-mates have big health problems now.'

K, another top athlete, played one of the most intensive sports in the world – squash – and once won the world junior title. But in the course of her career she had to go to more than 30 hospitals around the world, usually after a big tournament. She used oral steroids and nebulisers before a match, otherwise she would not have been able to play at all.

K embarked on a Buteyko course with a CP of about 10 seconds and the medication she took covered half the table, even after she had quit the sport that had been her life. After several weeks, when her medication was down to just one steroid tablet and one or no puffs of salbutamol, she began to practise squash again and was able to play with her mouth closed. (As a matter of fact, she taped her mouth shut with sticky tape, which looked rather peculiar but protected her from asthma.) She is now coming back into competitive squash, after an absence of four or five years, and even if she does not become a winner, she is already a winner – over her asthma.

What is the best sport for asthma?

So what is the best sport for asthma? There really is no 'best' sport, because what counts is not the sport, but your breath control. Some sports are more amenable than others to your efforts to control your breathing, however. Rhythmical exercise such as jogging, running, swimming, aerobics and cycling enable you to build up carbon dioxide through the activity of your muscles – while giving you the chance to slow down or stop to get your breath back.

By contrast, sports such as football and tennis, which involve sudden, erratic bursts of speed, make it harder for you to control your breathing.

One of the best sports for people with asthma is horse riding, because the physical bumping of your body against the horse as it trots 'breaks up' your breathing into fast and shallow rhythms, rather than the more dangerous deep breathing of some other sports.

One of the worst sports for asthma is chess – it is useless from the exercise point of view, and it induces hyperventilation.

Do's and don'ts of sport and asthma

- **Don't** use your puffer before sport. If you can't play sport without using your puffer, it means your body doesn't like it, recognises the danger and makes its protest through asthma. For the time being, it's better not to do sport at all. Once you have put an end to your asthma – which takes only a few days with the Buteyko method – then you can exercise without using salbutamol.
- **Do** breathe through your nose, keeping your mouth closed, whatever sport you undertake. Breathe only through your nose and if you feel that your need for breath is so great that you have to open your mouth to breathe, slow down or stop. The urge to open your mouth to breathe is a worrying sign: the next stage along this route may be an asthma attack.

  If you go swimming, ignore the standard advice to breathe in through your nose and out through your mouth. Instead, keep your mouth closed for breast stroke and back stroke, and for crawl, try to hold your face under water for four, six or even eight strokes.
- **Do** try to hold back your breathing after taking exercise. Remember, an asthma attack may happen only when you are breathing deeply. If you can control your breathing, you can control your asthma.

- **Do** check your control pause before and after sport. Then, instead of following the mantra that 'sport is good for asthma', you can measure how good each individual sport is for **your** asthma – or not, as the case may be. (It could of course have quite a different impact on somebody else.)

such as the nose, legs or anus – which may cause you nasal problems, varicose veins and/or haemorrhoids).

For the same reason – to conserve carbon dioxide – your body grows nasal polyps and develops blocked sinuses, which is why Professor Buteyko calls sinusitis 'asthma in the nose'. The symptoms of sinusitis which include mucus, swelling of the tissues, inability to breathe, even wheezing, are also symptoms suffered by people with asthma.

And just as with asthma, the standard medical treatments address only the symptoms, not the cause. As with asthma the treatments include steroids, as well as 'nose dilators' (as opposed to bronchodilators) in the form of nasal drops. But the treatment of nasal problems with chemical sprays only makes the problem worse.

This is because nasal sprays make the tissues (mucous membrane) inside your nose contract, but when the effect of the drug has worn off, your nose responds with a 'rebound' effect. In other words, your mucous membrane swells up more than ever before, so you spray more, swell up more, spray more – and so on, in a vicious circle of poor treatment.

How to unblock your nose without nasal sprays

This easy method takes only 20 or 30 seconds:

1. Breathe out normally.
2. Hold your breath, close your mouth and pinch your nose between two fingers.
3. When you can no longer comfortably hold your breath, let go of your nose – but keep your mouth closed and carry

CHAPTER EIGHT

Asthma and Your Nose

It has long been known that people with asthma often have nasal problems too, such as sinusitis, rhinitis, polyps or adenoids. Modern medicine often treats these associated problems surgically in the belief that removing the source of 'chronic infections' like these will restore normal breathing and improve asthma.

Unfortunately, many direct nasal treatments, such as the removal of polyps, bring only slight changes to health and it is well known that polyps almost always grow back again after surgery. This is because their roots are still there, not in the sinuses but in hyperventilation.

For polyps, like other nasal problems – and like asthma – are one of your body's defence mechanisms against overbreathing. Learn how to get rid of nasal problems and you will also learn how to get rid of asthma because these are two facets of the same problem.

What's more, if your doctors do manage to remove your polyps or clear your sinuses, your asthma is likely to get worse – because one of your defences against overbreathing has also been removed. Indeed, all people with nasal problems and asthma develop their nasal problems before their asthma, while many others go on to develop asthma after having polyps removed.

Look at the progress of this problem step by step, from your body's point of view:

1. You hyperventilate.
2. Your level of carbon dioxide goes down.
3. Your body reacts by causing your nose to become blocked.
4. You unblock your nose using a nasal spray.
5. Your body responds by making polyps in your nose.
6. Your polyps are surgically removed.
7. Your body grows new polyps.
8. The new polyps are surgically removed.
9. Your levels of carbon dioxide are still going down.
10. Your body responds with a new defence mechanism – asthma.

It follows that the more severe your nasal problems, the more severe your asthma is likely to be, because the bigger your problem of hyperventilation, the stronger your defence mechanisms are going to be too. The corollary is also true – that some people who have very strong bronchospasms don't have any nasal problems at all – because their bronchospasm is enough of a defence mechanism to make any other unnecessary.

Like the Four Horsemen of the Apocalypse, we ignore our bodies' messages at our peril. The First Horseman comes to block your nose – to tell you that you are hyperventilating. But you ignore him, open your mouth, use nasal drops; after all, everyone else breathes through their mouths, and your doctor hasn't told you not to.

So the Second Horseman visits you and gives you mild asthma or polyps – or both. What do you do? Out with the polyps; in with the bronchodilator drugs. Things could be better, but you feel all right.

Then the Third Horseman comes and he is really angry. His message is a serious one: you have got severe asthma. What do you do? You take your nebuliser, three times a day.

Finally, the fatal Fourth Horseman arrives – and that is the end of your story...

'Asthma in the nose'

Yet, as we have learned in this book, it doesn't have to be like that. With the Buteyko method, symptoms such as sinusitis and polyps will go away of their own accord, without surgery, when you have learned to recondition your breathing.

After two or three days of practising the Buteyko method your nasal passages will open up – and stay open. Polyps and sinusitis will disappear within a few weeks. Your doctor may shake his head and say this is impossible. But then he is unlikely to know much about the Buteyko method.

From a Buteyko point of view, sinusitis is one of your body's defence mechanisms against hyperventilation. To defend itself against the loss of carbon dioxide, your body constricts the arterial vessels which carry blood enriched by oxygen through areas such as the brain and the bronchial passages (this may cause you headaches and/or bronchospasm). Meanwhile your body also expands the venous vessels (which carry more carbon dioxide) to areas such as the nose, legs or anus – which may cause you nasal problems, varicose veins and/or haemorrhoids).

For the same reason – to conserve carbon dioxide – your body grows nasal polyps and develops blocked sinuses, which is why Professor Buteyko calls sinusitis 'asthma in the nose'. The symptoms of sinusitis which include mucus, swelling of the tissues, inability to breathe, even wheezing, are also symptoms suffered by people with asthma.

And just as with asthma, the standard medical treatments address only the symptoms, not the cause. As with asthma the treatments include steroids, as well as 'nose dilators' (as opposed to bronchodilators) in the form of nasal drops. But the treatment of nasal problems with chemical sprays only makes the problem worse.

This is because nasal sprays make the tissues (mucous membrane) inside your nose contract, but when the effect of the drug has worn off, your nose responds with a 'rebound' effect. In other words, your mucous membrane swells up more than ever before, so you spray more, swell up more, spray more – and so on, in a vicious circle of poor treatment.

How to unblock your nose without nasal sprays

This easy method takes only 20 or 30 seconds:

1. Breathe out normally.
2. Hold your breath, close your mouth and pinch your nose between two fingers.
3. When you can no longer comfortably hold your breath, let go of your nose – but keep your mouth closed and carry on breathing through your nose, which will now be 'open'.

Children and young people can do a dozen or more squats while pinching their noses, or they may walk upstairs while doing this exercise. Adults and elderly people can walk around the house, garden or office whole holding their breath, trying to take as many steps as they can.

Warning: If you start breathing through your mouth after this exercise – in other words hyperventilating – you may develop wheezing, coughing or even an asthma attack.

This simple exercise is not part of the Buteyko technique, but it does demonstrate the miraculous properties of breathing and carbon dioxide.

So what happened during this exercise? When you held your breath, you stopped losing carbon dioxide. The muscular exertion of doing squats or walking helped to increase your raised levels of carbon dioxide still further.

Before the exercise, your nose was blocked by expanded veins (caused by a shortage of carbon dioxide). Raising your levels of carbon dioxide made them return to their healthy, narrowed state – and your nose was unblocked.

This exercise will help your nose to stay unblocked for a few minutes or even hours, but eventually it will become blocked again because – unless you have changed your breathing pattern through the Buteyko technique – you are still hyperventilating and breathing out too much carbon dioxide.

The connection between too little carbon dioxide and a blocked nose is largely unknown to doctors. I once visited a hospital for children with asthma in Sydney, Australia. I met a nice man who was the head of the Respiratory Department there and we had a long discussion about hyperventilation, asthma and the Buteyko method. He asked me many intelligent questions and agreed with the theoretical part of Buteyko.

But then he said that he could not check how the method worked in his hospital because it entailed breathing through the nose, whereas practically all the children in his care breathed through their mouths – because their noses were blocked.

I told him that I could teach the children how to unblock their noses within a minute. He replied that in all the world's scientific literature there is no reference to the effects of carbon dioxide on a blocked nose. 'Sorry,' he told me. 'I'm very busy. Glad to have met you and have a nice day.'

Asthma and your tonsils

According to Professor Buteyko, nearly 90 per cent of children with asthma who are six years old or more should have their tonsils surgically removed. Tonsils are supposed to fight infections which are around us all the time. When an infection reaches the throat the battle begins; tonsils fight the infection, stopping it from getting any further down into our bodies. In the course of this battle, our tonsils often become large and painful, making it hard for us to swallow. This is a normal response and it is exactly what we should expect from our tonsils.

So why remove them? Surely we need our tonsils to prevent infections from reaching our lungs? These days it is far from easy to convince Ear, Nose and Throat specialists that our tonsils – as opposed to our adenoids or polyps – should be removed.

Unfortunately, most children with asthma no longer have healthy tonsils which will fight infection. Instead, their tonsils have shrunk. They remain small and they don't fight infection as they should. Tonsils like these are not painful, but they are no longer healthy, living tissues. According to Professor Buteyko, five to six years of hyperventilation (and if your child has asthma you can assume he or she has been hyperventilating for several years already) will 'kill' the tonsils.

But 'dead' tonsils are not harmlessly 'neutral'. On the contrary, they are poisonous to the rest of your body because they exude toxins into the bloodstream, suppressing your immune response. The smaller your tonsils are, the bigger concentraion of poison they have. Bad breath – more often attributed to a problem of the digestive system – is actually a sign of 'dead' tonsils, a typical smell of corpses.

Since the days of Jesus Christ and Lazarus no one has been able to revive corpses. It is equally impossible to restore 'dead' tonsils to health, so the only way to proceed is to remove them surgically. But beware: many doctors will try to persuade you to have the adenoids removed at the same time. Don't agree to this: adenoids are part of your defence mechanism and with the Buteyko method problems with adenoids will disappear.

After tonsillectomy, people often lose their pallor and regain a healthy colour. The tendency to go down with colds and flu diminishes. You will also find that – after the removal of tonsils – breathing becomes shallower too.

- **Don't** go to bed until you are really tired and when you can't do anything except sleep.
- **Don't** go to bed just because it is late. Wait until you really have to sleep.
- **Don't** go to bed during the day. If you have had a sleepless night which has left you feeling exhausted, just take a nap for 20 or 30 minutes while sitting up in a chair.
- **Do** make sure your mouth is closed when you sleep. If necessary, put sticky tape across your lips (see page 76). This may sound strange at first, but try it for one night and you will realise in the morning that this simple method helps to reduce phlegm, helps with snoring problems, provides a refreshing sleep – and helps prevent asthma attacks.

Doctors often argue that you cannot control hyperventilation while you are asleep. But with the Buteyko method, you can certainly control it during your waking hours and with these tips you can also reduce hyperventilation at night. Just as growing children learn how to wake up to go to the toilet rather than wetting their beds, so people trained in the Buteyko method develop a kind of guard mechanism which wakes them up when they start breathing too much.

Native American women used to use their fingers to make sure that the mouths of their children were closed when they were asleep, until their children developed the habit of breathing through their noses while asleep. Doctors of the time noted that these children were often healthier than their colonial contemporaries.

On the other side of the world, the Russian people of four centuries ago slept on short beds with high cushions

CHAPTER NINE

Asthma at Night

The fact that asthma gets worse at night and in the early morning has been known since this disease was first recognised. Moses Maimonides, who became physician to the Egyptian court, referred to what we would call nocturnal asthma in the 12th century.

The London physician Dr John Floyer wrote in 1698 about his own attacks of asthma: 'I have often observed the fit always to happen after sleep in the night.' Floyer's asthma attacks came on exclusively at night, every night, for seven long years!

In the 19th century, the distinguished Canadian doctor Sir William Osler wrote that 'nocturnal attacks are common. After a few hours of sleep the patient is aroused with a distressing sense of want of breath and a feeling of great oppression in the chest.'

Today's doctors describe the phenomenon of wheeziness in the small hours of the morning or on wakening as 'the morning dip' and regard this as one of the most characteristic features of asthma. As many as 80 per cent of people with asthma are thought to suffer nocturnal symptoms, yet modern medicine doesn't have an explanation for this.

However, Buteyko does offer an explanation for nocturnal asthma.

The Buteyko explanation

Asthma becomes worse at night and in the early hours of the morning because the horizontal position of your body during sleep increases hyperventilation. Professor Buteyko believes that this is because the natural position of our bodies is upright. We don't feel 'right' while standing on our heads; for related reasons, lying down flat is not the optimum position for our bodies' normal functions.

Contrary to the belief (common amongst doctors and scientists) that in sleep, our breathing is slow and shallow because little oxygen is required, your breathing gets deeper and deeper as you sleep. Watch a sleeping child with asthma and you will witness this change – or you may even hear it in the form of snoring. Or, wake yourself with your alarm clock during the night and you will discover for yourself that your breathing is deeper than during the day.

The truth is that when we are lying down, our breathing increases and so our levels of carbon dioxide go down. Our bodies respond by trying to retain carbon dioxide, using the defence mechanisms of phlegm and bronchoconstriction. This is why people with asthma often wake up with problems of phlegm, wheezing, tightness in the chest – or with an asthma attack.

Not surprisingly, then, the worst time for asthma is during the small hours, especially between four and six in the morning, the hours when the death rate from asthma is at its highest.

POSITIONS FOR BREATHING

- The vertical position is **best** for breathing. Sitting up in a chair may make it difficult to sleep, but this position should be used at times when your asthma symptoms are bad. Some severe asthmatics have discovered this for themselves in the fight for breath which makes it impossible to lie down.
- Lying on your back and breathing through your mouth is the **worst** way to sleep.
- While sleeping in bed, Professor Buteyko has observed that it is best to lie on your left hand side with your mouth closed and with your knees pulled up to your chest (the foetal position). He believes that, ideally, children should sleep on their tummies.
- Buteyko practitioners have observed that sleeping on your right hand side is not as bad for breathing as sleeping on your back – but not as good as sleeping on your left side.

Helping you get through the night

Buteyko practitioners have observed that people with asthma have a better quality of sleep if they sleep on a hard bed (such as a futon) with a thin mattress. Sleeping with a high pile of pillows under your head and shoulders may also help.

Professor Buteyko also recommends that people with asthma should sleep less and deeply, rather than more and with dreams. How short should your sleep be? The shorter the better. If you can manage on four hours a night, very good. If you can manage on two, so much the better. If you can't face having so little sleep, then just do your best.

- **Don't** go to bed until you are really tired and when you can't do anything except sleep.
- **Don't** go to bed just because it is late. Wait until you really have to sleep.
- **Don't** go to bed during the day. If you have had a sleepless night which has left you feeling exhausted, just take a nap for 20 or 30 minutes while sitting up in a chair.
- **Do** make sure your mouth is closed when you sleep. If necessary, put sticky tape across your lips (see page 76). This may sound strange at first, but try it for one night and you will realise in the morning that this simple method helps to reduce phlegm, helps with snoring problems, provides a refreshing sleep – and helps prevent asthma attacks.

Doctors often argue that you cannot control hyperventilation while you are asleep. But with the Buteyko method, you can certainly control it during your waking hours and with these tips you can also reduce hyperventilation at night. Just as growing children learn how to wake up to go to the toilet rather than wetting their beds, so people trained in the Buteyko method develop a kind of guard mechanism which wakes them up when they start breathing too much.

Native American women used to use their fingers to make sure that the mouths of their children were closed when they were asleep, until their children developed the habit of breathing through their noses while asleep. Doctors of the time noted that these children were often healthier than their colonial contemporaries.

On the other side of the world, the Russian people of four centuries ago slept on short beds with high cushions in the belief that if they lay down flat, their spirit – which in Russian means much the same as 'breath' – might leave their bodies.

Professor Buteyko points out that nearly all animals and birds sleep with their noses or beaks under a paw or wing, knowing instinctively that this is a way to retain more carbon dioxide. Young children who sleep in the 'praying position' with their face in their pillows are doing the same thing, but in Western culture we are unfortunately in the habit of turning children over.

A NIGHT-TIME TIP

Another useful tip for people who regularly suffer asthma attacks at night is to break up your sleep by setting your alarm clock. The point of this is to stop hyperventilation.

1. Plan to wake yourself an hour to an hour and a half before the usual time of your asthma attack. You are going to be woken by asthma symptoms anyway, so you have nothing to lose. Better to be woken by an alarm clock than by an asthma attack!

2. Sit up in your bed. This is important because sitting up helps you to control your breathing.

3. Breathe gently for a few minutes until you feel that your breathing has normalised and that you have calmed down.

4. Lie down quietly and fall asleep, having successfully avoided an asthma attack.

To sum up...

- Sleep less
- Go to bed only when you are really sleepy

- Never sleep on your back, but on your left hand side or on your stomach.
- Sleep with your mouth closed, taping it if necessary.
- Use the 'broken sleep' method when your asthma is bad, and/or sleep in a chair.

CHAPTER TEN

Asthma and Allergy

An allergy is an adverse immune system reaction to a substance that most people find harmless. Allergies can manifest themselves in a number of ways, from headache, sneezing, watery eyes to stuffed sinuses or fatigue – and obviously they can trigger an asthma attack. So why should your immune system be different from, say, your husband's? Why do you cough and sneeze from the smell of cut grass in your back yard, when your husband actually cut it and feels nothing?

The answer lies in understanding that having a strong immune system means having a normal acid-alkaline balance (otherwise known as pH level) in the body. You can break this delicate balance so easily if you over-breathe. You exhale too much carbon dioxide and, because carbon dioxide is acidic, your body's interior environment becomes too alkaline. Normal immune reactions become allergic reactions.

Hyperventilation can shift your acid/alkaline balance within one or two minutes – but you can restore it using the Buteyko Method.

Allergy is not the **cause** of asthma (see page 140–1), but it is certainly one of the major **triggers** which may bring on asthma symptoms. Dust mites, cats, dogs, horses, red wine, white bread, petrol, perfume, cut grass, cigarette smoke, pollution: the list of potential allergens which can trigger asthma goes on and on...

But why is it that some people will suffer from asthma symptoms when they come into contact with these allergens, whereas others can drink, smoke, eat whatever they want and enjoy life free of symptoms? To deal with allergy we have to understand why this unusual sensitivity is possessed by some people and not others.

The usual medical advice given to people with allergies is to avoid the allergens which induce their allergic symptoms. Sometimes this can be simple: if you know that red wine makes you feel ill, you can drink white wine instead. But often things are not so straightforward. It's not always possible to avoid all the allergens which affect you – and even if you do, other allergens may appear. **For avoiding allergens does not eliminate the cause of allergy**. It reminds me of the story of the boy who was allergic to so many things that he had to live in a protective suit and helmet like an astronaut, and breathe artificial air. He was protected from his trigger factors, but he still had his allergy!

The Buteyko view of allergy

Professor Buteyko addresses the problem of allergy from a different perspective. He explains allergy as an imbalance of your immune system and of the metabolic processes of your body. This is caused by lack of carbon dioxide which – as we have seen – is a result of hyperventilation. It is not the dust mites or animals which trigger your asthma symp-

A RUSSIAN TALE

The famous Moscow Circus artist Kuklachev used to work with many cats in a show called 'Cat House'. Unfortunately, he was so allergic to cats that whenever he approached them he started to sneeze and his skin became itchy. Because cats were important to his way of making a living, and because his job took him all around the world, he tried a wide range of remedies to get rid of his allergies – to no avail. Professors from many different countries told him the only thing he could do was to get rid of his cats.

Finally, when he realised that Professor Buteyko treated more than simply asthma, he asked him for help and received treatment.

Two weeks later Kuklachev was on television with his cats who were climbing on his head and shoulders – and yet he showed no signs of allergy. 'Look what Professor Buteyko did for me!' he said. 'I have no signs of allergy whatsoever. I have visited Professors in Switzerland, Israel and America, only to find the cure for my allergy here in Moscow!'

Since then, all of Russia has known that Professor Buteyko treats allergies too.

toms which are the **cause** of allergy. It is your immune system's inability to protect you from these and millions of other potential trigger factors in everyday life which is at the root of the problem.

Hyperventilation causes the reactions of your immune system to become abnormal – in other words you react allergically. But the opposite is also true: as long as your immune system is strong enough, you will not have any allergic reactions – whatever you come into contact with, from cats to French perfume. The Buteyko method normalises your immune system which has been weakened by hyperventilation.

Allergy – a world problem

Other than avoidance, modern medicine does have one rather controversial method of 'treating' allergy. This method, called hyposensitisation, is in a sense the opposite of the avoidance strategy. It involves injecting you with micro-doses of the allergen which affects you in the hope that this will 'educate' your immune system to produce the antibodies needed to fight this foreign substance. This treatment can go on for many years – but it may have few, if any positive results. This is because your immune system is suppressed by hyperventilation, and hyposensitisation is not going to boost your immune system, which remains unable to deal with allergens.

Moreover, because allergic people are usually allergic to quite a few things, even if you get rid of the reaction to one allergen, you are liable to develop a new allergic reaction to something else – even, perhaps, to your hyposensitisation treatment.

Doctors know, or are supposed to know, the danger of this treatment. P. Brisco, author of *Asthma: Questions You Have, Answers You Need* (1997), writes: 'Desensitisation is dangerous 'because it involves deliberately injecting a substance to which the patient is known to be severely allergic. This can promote severe and dangerous reactions. Formerly there were regular deaths from this procedure and for a time it was completely abandoned in Britain.'

Yet some doctors have resumed this treatment, believing it can reduce the amount of drugs a patient needs. Lists of the delayed reactions (which can occur from four to 24 hours after the injection) include headache, fever, lethargy, or some wheezing. Should you experience these delayed reactions – or a lengthy reaction – you are advised to contact your doctor or go to a hospital casualty department immediately.

The severe reactions which can follow desensitisation treatment are:

>...chest tightness and a full-blown asthma attack, exceptional difficulty in breathing, hives, stomach pains, pains, difficulty in swallowing, fainting and nausea. An adrenaline injection, antihistamines and theophylline may be needed to stop a systemic reaction from progressing to anaphylaxis, or anaphylactic shock, a severe and sometimes fatal systemic reaction.
>
>Although deaths from allergy to injections are rare, most of them involve anaphylaxis and lack of resuscitation equipment in the doctor's surgery. For that reason, allergy injections should be administered only in a doctor's surgery where facilities and trained personnel are available to treat life-threatening reaction.

SIMON, AGED 36

The course has been of great interest and benefit. There is no doubt that the Buteyko method makes a difference, though I hope I have the determination to keep up the programme.

Even after all this, writes Brisco, 'no cure for asthma has yet been found...Some doctors call desensitisation an inexact, controversial and dangerous therapy because they don't know in advance whether someone with asthma will benefit from a lengthy series of injections. But other doctors are enthusiastic about desensitisation.'

How can it be that some doctors remain enthusiastic? The American doctor K.A. Lasko, in his book *The Great Billion Dollar Medical Swindle* puts forward this theory:

> These treatments, these weekly shots, these exposures to the thing you cannot tolerate, cost the patient every week. Sometimes the allergic condition actually gets better. Temporarily . . . Fortunately for the allergist, his patients are rarely, if ever, cured. They must keep coming back year after year, week after week. For a shot, for a fee, for what?

In the UK and other countries with a national health service it may not be the individual patient's money that is being wasted, but this is still an unnecessary and costly treatment. It can go on for as long as five years. Compare this with a five-day Buteyko treatment programme, after which you can reduce the amount of medication needed to control asthma to a tenth of the former level.

Asthma triggered by allergy – first line of defence

It is well known that certain foods, smell, drinks, etc can trigger an asthma attack, and people have been rushed to intensive care or even died after eating dried apricots, nuts or chocolate, drinking red wine or a fizzy drink, smelling cats, horses or cut grass – or many other things. (Hay fever, by the way, was first 'discovered' – described – by a sixteenth-century doctor who noticed that he sneezed and cried after smelling fresh roses.) So what do you do if, say, you have accidentally eaten something which you know will lead to an asthma attack in a few minutes? Alternative treatments cannot give immediate relief in this instance: you need help now, this minute, and I would strongly recommend that you use a conventional medicine such as an anti-histamine.

Or, exercise using the Buteyko Method.

1. Sit down.
2. Breathe out.
3. Hold your breath for five seconds (count slowly 1-2-3-4-5).
4. Inhale through your nose as gently as you can.
5. Exhale through your nose and hold your breath for ten seconds (again, count slowly).
6. Inhale gently through your nose.
7. Exhale for a count of 15.
8. Inhale through your nose and start breathing as shallowly as you can for five minutes. This should increase your carbon dioxide levels, which will restore acid-based equilibrium, which will stop the allergic reaction, which will stop the asthma attack, while will make you feel happy. . .

If this exercise does not bring relief within five minutes, take the medication which normally helps you, and learn the Buteyko Method so that you can do the exercise more effectively next time!

To give one example, I was once having dinner in a Turkish restaurant with a lady who suffered from many allergies and was exceptionally careful in choosing her food – no bread, no red wine, no spinach, no yeast. She could eat almost nothing. But her rice must have been dusted with some flour or additive – and the moment she tried it she developed a reaction. Her breathing got very deep, her chest began to move up and down as if she had been for a good run, she became breathless and very scared.

I said to her, ' Put your hand on your chest and suppress your breathing.'

She tried, but said, 'I can't do it!'

I said, 'Try not to move your hand. Hold your breath, count inside, 1-2-3, then breathe in, breathe out, count 1-2-3-4-5, and so on.'

We did it together and after 15–20 minutes, when she was breathing out for a count of 40, she was OK. It was good that she came on a Buteyko course the very next day – even I can't teach the Buteyko Method in 20 minutes, and nobody can learn it that fast!

I forgot to mention, that that lady would normally have used eight to ten puffs of Salbutamol to stop an asthma attack brought on by food.

Some practical applications of the Buteyko method and allergy

Asthmatics frequently develop asthma symptoms when they happen to be in a smoky bar, in a home where there are cats, dogs or birds, in a garden with freshly cut grass or in a yard where horses are kept. Also, up to 80 per cent of them (asthmatics, not horses) experience wheezing, coughing, tightness in the chest or nasal problems when there is a sharp change in the weather – when they go out into the cold street from a warm building, or vice versa.

All these situations normally require 'puffers' or bronchodilators, but this necessity can easily be avoided with these simple breathing techniques:

• When you are passing through a bar, garden, etc or when you come in from or go out into the cold:

1. Breathe out.
2. Hold your breath.
3. Take 10–15 steps without breathing.
4. Stop and breathe very shallowly for 20–30 seconds.
5. Walk on, breathing gently and shallowly until you reach a 'safe' place.

This technique can also be used when you are crossing a road with lots of car exhaust, walking through the perfume department in a shop, and so on.

• When you can't just pass through the 'danger area' i.e. if you are spending the evening in a bar, visiting friends who have pets, cutting the grass yourself or stuck on a train or bus with lots of flu viruses around:

1. Breathe out and hold your breath for as long as you can.
2. Start breathing very shallowly.
3. Try not to talk. This may not be much fun if you are enjoying a social evening with friends, but even in these cir-

cumstances you should be conscious of what you are doing and make an effort to talk less than usual – otherwise it will not be possible to control your breath.

Why does it work? Because by breathing shallowly you inhale two, three, even five times fewer allergens, irritants, pollutants or viruses. And because by breathing shallowly you raise the defensive capabilities of your immune system.

Raising your control pause

The control pause is a measure of your hyperventilation and asthma, and it is a mistake to try to increase it by holding your breath longer. A high CP – of 60 seconds or more – is the ultimate goal of the Buteyko method (and every asthmatic). But attempts to increase it by extending breath-holding beyond the point of the first discomfort are meaningless – a bit like using inaccurate scales in the hope of losing weight. You can practise and achieve better readings in your peak flow meter or CP; you can learn how to deceive your friends/enemies/doctors and even yourself into thinking your asthma is better – but you can't deceive your asthma.

So how do you raise your CP? Because it is a measure of your breathing, it goes up as a result of: breathing less frequently and more shallowly; physical exercise; an active lifestyle; taking the correct dose of medication; and minimizing mistakes which make you breathe more deeply – overeating, oversleeping and, of course, most seriously, overbreathing.

At the moment there is (as far as I know) no method, treatment, trick or technique apart from the Buteyko method which aims to make your breathing shallower and does this directly and consistently. Even meditation, yoga, t'ai-chi, relaxation – all of which can make you breathe less – do it for a short time (when you are meditating or performing the exercises), but indirectly, with no measure of the progress. And, of course, none of these treatments embraces all the possible problems facing asthmatics. But in the Buteyko method of treating hyperventilation – and incidentally asthma, allergy, eczema, sinusitis, hay fever, insomnia, panic attacks, heart disorders and many other complaints – the control pause is a precise measurement of hyperventilation, carbon dioxide level and, ultimately, health. That's why it is so important to check it correctly and not to repeat the common mistake of overstretching it.

The control pause shows your current condition and helps to prevent your asthma deteriorating. That's why it makes sense to check it several times a day– after meals, after sleep, sport, meetings, long talks, etc – and if you find that your control pause has gone down you have to be very aware of your asthma. Buteyko is absolutely clear on this point: **you can have an asthma problem only if your CP is low, which means you are breathing too deeply**. You cannot have an asthma problem if your CP is high.

WHEEZY BRONCHITIS – OR ASTHMA?

Many people with bronchitis also have a wheeze, and this combination tends to confuse doctors. What is it, they wonder – asthma, or just 'wheezy bronchitis'?

These days – in contrast to forty odd years ago – doctors tend to treat children with 'wheezy bronchitis' as if they have asthma. (In the past, doctors thought the term asthma might alarm parents and so usually avoided it. In any case, treatment for asthma was at that stage not very 'advanced'.)

As a consequence of the confusion surrounding this diagnosis today, children with what was formerly known as 'wheezy bronchitis' (bronchitis with mucus which produces a wheezy cough) are often prescribed asthma drugs. Within a few weeks they become real asthmatics because their medication has made them hyperventilate even more than before.

So what should you do if your child develops a wheeze? Professor Buteyko recommends that you don't try to get rid of the wheeze artificially with drugs or herbal remedies – or your child will end up developing asthma as the next available defence mechanism against hyperventilation.

Instead, decrease your child's breathing using Buteyko techniques and the wheeze will disappear by itself. Be reassured that the wheeze in itself is not dangerous: it is merely the audible signal of your child's body that all is not well. Only in emergencies and/or when your child is experiencing obvious breathing difficulties should you give your child asthma medication.

Conversely, according to Professor Buteyko, children with asthma may develop bronchitis as a result of regular inhalation of cromoglycate drugs (see page 101).

CHAPTER ELEVEN

Asthma and Diet

Your diet can be an important factor when it comes to asthma – especially considerations of **when** you eat, and the **way** you eat. There are also some types of food that can make your asthma very much worse.

However, when thinking about your diet, do remember that asthma is essentially a breathing disorder, not an eating disorder. Breathing is more immediately vital to us: you can survive for weeks without food, but only for a few minutes without breathing. Buteyko practitioners never discuss issues of food or diet with their patients until they are two or three days into a Buteyko course – which means they have already experienced significant improvement in their asthma from learning how to reduce hyperventilation.

The Buteyko view of diet

There is one very simple and natural rule at the heart of the Buteyko philosophy of food, and that is **eat when you are hungry – and only when you are hungry**. If you are not hungry, do not eat. The reason for this is that if you eat when you are not hungry, your hyperventilation will increase, making your asthma symptoms worse. There is only one situation in which you really **must** eat, and that is if you have hypoglycaemia and your blood sugar level drops.

We have all been told at times, 'You must eat your breakfast' or 'You must eat to get energy'. But forget these exhortations because they do you no good. Your body will tell you when you need to eat: not your husband or your wife, your father or your mother, not a dietician or a diet book, but your own body.

We are even told, 'You must eat because you are sick.' Yet no animal will touch food when it is sick. Some people say they eat breakfast because they are told they must take their medication in the morning 'after food'. But if you are not hungry it is better to take your medicine and then drink a glass of water or juice, or have a cup of tea.

In the same mistaken tradition, parents often say to their children, 'You must eat if you want to grow big', but what they really mean is 'You must eat because I feel better when you eat.' Parents sometimes say to me, 'My son doesn't eat at all, and if I didn't push him to eat he wouldn't eat anything.' Or they say, 'He's never hungry' – but children learn to hate eating if they are always pushed to eat. Some parents run the risk of making themselves feel better – but their children worse – by making their children eat!

No one can survive without food and when children are really hungry they will eat. Offer them healthy food – no junk food – and wait until they are ready to eat it. If you push them to eat, you will suppress their natural appetite and disturb their delicate metabolic processes.

Don't eat 'upfront' if you are not hungry. Having breakfast before you go to work – or making your child eat

BUTEYKO'S RULES ON FOOD

- Eat only when you are hungry.
- Do not overeat.
- Avoid high-protein foods.
- Avoid caffeine (chocolate, coffee, strong tea).
- Avoid milk – any milk, including goats' milk or soya milk, because of their high protein content.
- Eat plenty of fresh green vegetables and whole grains.
- Use natural sea salt, not 'table salt'.
- Drink water when you are thirsty – and only when you are thirsty.
- **The only 'good' food is the food you eat when you are hungry.**

before going out – is not a good idea. It is better to give your child a banana or a sandwich to eat later in the day, or to take a snack with you to the office. People say, 'If I don't eat breakfast I will be hungry later', but a day is a long time and you don't know how you are going to feel later.

Simply eat at any time when you are hungry. This means that your body is ready for food, and it will digest food much more easily when you are hungry than when you are not. If you wake up in the middle of the night because you are hungry, get up and have something to eat. Forget the rules about breakfast, lunch and dinner: forget about calories. **The issue here is not that overeating gives you too many calories, but that overeating makes you hyperventilate.**

Think back to when you last ate a big lunch or dinner. Didn't you feel breathless afterwards? And bear in mind that if you are not hungry, any eating is overeating. So put aside that diet sheet you were given by your dietician or naturopath. You may not **want** to eat as much as they have outlined for you at breakfast or at lunchtime. So don't.

Bear in mind too that while the Buteyko method is essentially a technique for retraining your breathing, many people automatically lose weight when they stop hyperventilating because for the first time in many years their metabolism has begun to function normally.

So eat as often as you want to, but only when you are . . . what? Yes, **hungry!**

'Good' foods and 'bad' foods

There are some kinds of food which, according to Professor Buteyko's observations, can increase your hyperventilation. These include the high-protein foods such as eggs, cheese, cottage cheese and, worst of all, fish.

Food and drinks which contain caffeine – such as chocolate, cocoa, tea, coffee and colas – should also be avoided because they increase hyperventilation, although the odd cup of tea or coffee won't hurt. If you are worried about giving up milk because of the risks of osteoporosis, or because you believe your child should be getting plenty of calcium, there are numerous other sources of this mineral. Of course, if you are allergic to any kind of food, avoid it, until you have been trained in the Buteyko method.

According to Professor Buteyko the foods that should form the basis of your diet are the usual green vegetables, other fresh vegetables (but not too many potatoes) and whole grains such as brown rice.

Professor Buteyko also advocates we eat more spices such as black pepper, mustard and sea salt – as well as more onions and garlic.

Salt is good for you if it is sea salt and useless – or even harmful – if it is 'table salt'. This is because sea salt contains many micro-elements and minerals. Professor Buteyko recommends that you should use sea salt for cooking and as a natural remedy for palpitations, coughs and headaches. Just put a teaspoon of sea salt in a glass of hot water, stir and drink. You should feel relief from your symptoms after 10 or 15 minutes.

In the west we have been encouraged to eat plenty of fruit, but Professor Buteyko recommends that you don't overdo it. Some fruits – such as oranges and strawberries – can cause allergic reactions in some people. If this is a problem with you, get your vitamins from vegetables instead.

Professor Buteyko also believes we should drink as much (or as little) water as we want, depending on whether we are thirsty or not. If you are thirsty, drink until your thirst is satisfied. If you are not thirsty, don't drink at all. Current notions that it is good for us to drink some eight glasses of water a day are not proven. As with food, it is better to listen to your body, which will tell you how much you need to drink.

Professor Buteyko also says that the best drinking water is made from melted ice, for complex reasons to do with the crystalline structure of water. Make ice in your own freezer, then let it melt, drink – and you will notice the difference for yourself!

3. Poor oxygenation leads to hypoxia and a whole gamut of medical disorders.
4. CO_2 is a smooth muscle vessel dilator. Therefore a shortfall of CO_2 causes spasming of brain tissue, bronchus tissue etc.
5. Hyperventilation causes a progressive loss of CO_2. The higher the breathing, the lower the CO_2 level.
6. CO_2 is the catalyst to the body's metabolic processes, playing a vital role in biosynthesis of amino acids and their amides, Lipids, Carbohydrates, etc. This is explained in more detail in "The Biochemical Basis of K.P. Buteyko's Theory of the Disease of Deep Respiration".

Through an understanding of current physiology we should begin to see the links between CO_2 and oxygenation of the body, CO_2 and disease. It is clear that a deepening of the breathing does not mean an increase in oxygen uptake. On the contrary it means a decrease in oxygenation, which leads to hypoxia, imbalance in the acid-alkali balance, and cell spasming.

The fifth point of physiological understanding explains the destructively poisonous influence that hyperventilation has on the organism. It shows us clearly (in conjunction with the other points) that over-breathing leads to imbalance in the body and general deterioration of health.

The Dangers Of Hyperventilation

The term "hyperventilation" should be clearly defined. It is not reserved only to the most extreme and visible cases. Hyperventilation simply means "an increase in the function of the lungs above the normal recommended amount." The significance of Buteyko's discoveries hinge on the diagnosis of what Buteyko termed "hidden hyperventilation", that is long term over-breathing that is not clearly visible in the patient.

If a patient hyperventilating 30 Lt/min. can receive disastrous physical repercussions in the very short term, then it should be understood that over-breathing 5-10 Lt/min will have equally dire consequences over the long term. The average asthmatic over-breathes between 3 to 5 times the recommended amount, sometimes more.

The detrimental influence of the deep breathing on the organism is a direct result of the creation of a CO_2 deficit. This has been proven by many experiments, starting with the work of the well-known physiologist, Dr D Henderson, in 1909. In his experiments, animals were mechanically induced to deep breath and died as a result.

Acid-Alkali Balance

Through its conversion into carbonic acid, CO_2 is the most vital player in the maintaining of the body's acid-base balance. Lowering CO_2 in the

CHAPTER TWELVE

Asthma and Your Child

Earlier in this book we saw how many of the conventional medical approaches to asthma simply don't work because they fail to address the fundamental cause of asthma which is overbreathing. It follows that conventional medicine will have many 'solutions' to your child's asthma that are in fact useless – or even harmful.

In this chapter we look at how the Buteyko method can help your child overcome the frightening and upsetting symptoms of asthma, while for the most part steering clear of drugs.

An inherited problem?

We're all aware that asthma tends to run in families. The evidence points to the fact that there is an 'asthma gene' – or several genes – in 20 to 30 per cent of people, which determines whether or not you will have a predisposition to asthma. Fortunately, this is no more than a predisposition which may or may not result in asthma.

The conventional medical view is that when people with this gene (or genes) come into contact with an 'environmental trigger', asthma is the result. The Buteyko point of view is different, in that we see hyperventilation as the root cause of breathing problems in those susceptible people who develop symptoms of asthma.

According to Professor Buteyko, up to 50 per cent of children in families where one parent is asthmatic may develop asthma. The figure goes up to 90 per cent in families where both parents are asthmatic. His view is that newborn children do not have asthma, but that they may develop asthma after a few months of hyperventilation.

However, the Buteyko method can stop your child's asthma, whatever his or her genetic inheritance, by tackling the basic problem of overbreathing.

Starting in the womb: asthma and pregnancy

If you are a pregnant woman with asthma, you may find that your asthma symptoms improve during pregnancy – or, unfortunately, you may find the reverse. There is no hard and fast rule about how asthma affects pregnant women: some feel better, some feel worse, others feel no difference at all.

What is clear, however, is that it is possible to prevent asthma problems from developing in your unborn baby using Buteyko techniques. Nature has established a perfect but delicate balance of carbon dioxide and oxygen in the womb which ensures that the foetus does not become ill. The level of carbon dioxide in the womb is in fact twice as high as the post-natal level, while the level of oxygen is five times less than after birth.

Hyperventilation in the mother can break this delicate balance, causing – according to Professor Buteyko – a range of health problems. He argues that if you over-breathe, the oxygen available to the baby becomes less, resulting in problems that may be as serious as miscarriage.

While many women find that focusing on their breathing can be of help during labour, it is important to avoid any 'deep breathing' exercises during pregnancy and birth which will increase hyperventilation. Professor Buteyko's view is that – rather than deep breathing – it is shallow, controlled, nasal breathing that can decrease pain in labour because higher carbon dioxide levels in the blood relax the muscles.

When the baby of a woman who has been habitually hyperventilating emerges into the world, the baby too may start life by hyperventilating. She doesn't yet have asthma, but in as little as four months, she may start to show the first signs of this disease.

And as explained elsewhere in this book, the remedies are straightforward. Make sure that her mouth stays closed to reduce hyperventilation, and do not overfeed her. Should she need to take asthma medicines, avoid using a nebuliser on a regular basis: use it strictly according to need and for as short a time as possible. Better still, use a spacer (a device to help infants inhale asthma medications) rather than a nebuliser.

Once upon a time: a sad children's story...

The story of what happens to a typical child with asthma who is treated with conventional medicine rarely makes for happy reading. It all begins when the child is still in the womb. Because his mother has been overbreathing, her baby develops oxygen deficiency. When he is born he may

WHEEZY BRONCHITIS – OR ASTHMA?

Many people with bronchitis also have a wheeze, and this combination tends to confuse doctors. What is it, they wonder – asthma, or just 'wheezy bronchitis'?

These days – in contrast to forty odd years ago – doctors tend to treat children with 'wheezy bronchitis' as if they have asthma. (In the past, doctors thought the term asthma might alarm parents and so usually avoided it. In any case, treatment for asthma was at that stage not very 'advanced'.)

As a consequence of the confusion surrounding this diagnosis today, children with what was formerly known as 'wheezy bronchitis' (bronchitis with mucus which produces a wheezy cough) are often prescribed asthma drugs. Within a few weeks they become real asthmatics because their medication has made them hyperventilate even more than before.

So what should you do if your child develops a wheeze? Professor Buteyko recommends that you don't try to get rid of the wheeze artificially with drugs or herbal remedies – or your child will end up developing asthma as the next available defence mechanism against hyperventilation.

Instead, decrease your child's breathing using Buteyko techniques and the wheeze will disappear by itself. Be reassured that the wheeze in itself is not dangerous: it is merely the audible signal of your child's body that all is not well. Only in emergencies and/or when your child is experiencing obvious breathing difficulties should you give your child asthma medication.

Conversely, according to Professor Buteyko, children with asthma may develop bronchitis as a result of regular inhalation of cromoglycate drugs (see page 101).

be put in an oxygen chamber to 'remedy' this problem, but as we have seen (page 108), this 'solution' only makes the symptoms worse. As pure oxygen is known to 'burn' the lungs – even of adults – this baby is already on the road to developing breathing problems in the future.

After birth, too, there are further factors which contribute to overbreathing in babies, such as mouth breathing and overfeeding – not to mention the radically changed environment. The baby has left the safety of the high carbon dioxide womb for an atmosphere which has far higher levels of oxygen (20 per cent) in proportion to carbon dioxide (0.03 per cent).

If the baby should develop a wheeze, the doctor may prescribe bronchodilators – to be administered through a nebuliser three times a day, regardless of the baby's condition. This means more hyperventilation for the child – and a yet higher chance of developing asthma.

But life goes on, and the baby becomes a child who can use a cromoglycate drug through an inhaler. (Alternatively, he may be put on a nebuliser or spacer with a pressurised inhaler.) By the time this little boy goes to school, he should be able to use a drug powder inhaler or autohaler. By now, he may have developed bronchitis as a result of the cromoglycate drugs which are very damaging to the bronchi.

By now our little boy has asthma and bronchitis and takes bronchodilators and steroids regularly, according to a timetable rather than according to need. This is in spite of the fact that bronchodilators increase hyperventilation (the cause of the asthma), and in spite of the fact that too many steroids cause the suppression of the body's own natural steroids.

Meanwhile, everyone from sports coaches to teachers to physiotherapists – even doctors – is incorrectly teaching the little boy that deep breathing is good for him – instead of teaching him that he should close his mouth, breathe through his nose and avoid overbreathing.

He may also be taking medicines or herbal remedies to try to get rid of the phlegm caused by his bronchitis. Or he may be simply trying to cough it up. Either way, he will be making his hyperventilation problem worse. And whether he coughs or takes medicines, the phlegm will still be there again in the morning, trying to protect him from further loss of carbon dioxide.

Now his doctor decides the time for stronger medicines has come and so our little boy is prescribed a long-acting bronchodilator which keeps his bronchotubes open for twelve hours at a stretch. The result is even greater hyperventilation, even worse asthma – and so the round of nebulisers, hospitals and massive doses of steroids begins. In hospital they may put him on the nebuliser every hour (despite the fact the nebulisers have been linked to the deaths of thousands of people in New Zealand during the 1980s). He is also likely to be given oxygen in hospital, again adding to his asthma problems. In addition, the huge doses of steroids given to him in hospital have made him moon faced.

After being discharged from hospital he is put on a regime of nebulisers and oral steroids. But because the bronchodilator drugs in nebulisers increase hyperventilation while steroids decrease it, this is rather like being given medicine for diarrhoea and constipation at the same time. The mechanism which regulates his breathing is now thoroughly confused.

His steroids have been prescribed for five days only – regardless of his individual needs, although he must stay on the bronchodilator drugs. The result is that in a few weeks' time, when the effects of the steroids finally wear off, his condition deteriorates. He has another severe asthma attack. The ambulance is called and it's back to the hospital again for more oxygen, more nebulisers, more steroids – and so on in a vicious circle of ever-worsening asthma.

For most modern children to date, this has been a story without a happy ending. Now however, the Buteyko method offers an alternative: a healthy life free of asthma symptoms and free of drugs.

Stopping asthma in your child

In conclusion, there are a number of practical day to day steps that you can take to stop your child becoming ill with asthma:

- Teach your child to keep his or her mouth closed, reducing hyperventilation. Ask your child's teacher to remind him while at school.
- Make sure your child remembers to take preventive medicines (steroids) before going to school. Children don't see the immediate benefit of taking these medicines, so they tend to think they're not important.
- Your child should always have a puffer in his school bag or pocket to use when he can't breathe.
- Teach your child to use reliever medicines ('puffers') only when needed, one puff at a time.
- Your child should not play sport if he needs to use an

inhaler first. After a Buteyko workshop, he will be able to play any sport without using reliever medicines first.

- Let the school know that you don't want your child to be put on a nebuliser except in an extreme situation – for instance, when he is still in difficulties after three puffs of reliever medicine. This is in fact an emergency, and you should hurry to take your child home, give him steroids and take him to a good doctor who will not put him on a nebuliser three times a day.

- Children as young as three are capable of taking reliever medicine through a puffer, which is preferable to a nebuliser which dispenses much larger doses of bronchodilator medicine (50 times more, in fact: one puff of the average bronchodilator gives 100 mcg, while a dose of nebuliser is 5 mg). And because 'delivery' is more efficient through a nebuliser, the effects may be even more powerful. But for infants who really need a dose of reliever medicine, just a few seconds on a nebuliser may be necessary.

- Make sure that you explain all you know about asthma to your child. Some children treat puffers as toys, passing them around the playground whether or not they have asthma. If they understood more about asthma, perhaps they wouldn't.

- Teach your child how to remedy a blocked nose by pinching his nose and holding his breath (see page 126).

- Enrol your child in a Buteyko workshop, and practise the Buteyko method.

Theoretical Understanding behind the Buteyko Technique

The Buteyko technique represents a development of the hyper-ventilation syndrome theory. This theory is based on the contemporary understanding of the immense biological role of the carbon dioxide gas in the human organism.

The human metabolism developed in the ancient geological eras when carbon dioxide in the air and water was represented in tens of percent. It is probably due to this factor that a definite concentration of CO_2 (7% approx.) must be an absolutely essential condition of each human cell in order for it to sustain all the normal pathways of the biochemical processes.

The problem faced by the evolving human organism has been the depletion of CO_2 in our atmosphere from the tens of percent of ancient eras to the current level (1982) of 0.03%. Human evolution has dealt with this dilemma by creating an autonomous internal air environment within the alveolar spaces of the lungs. These alveoli contain around 6.5% of CO_2, quite a contrast to the surrounding air. The gaseous mix in the womb is also an interesting indicator of the ideal human environment. Here there exists between 7 to 8% of CO_2. Professor Buteyko was asked to speak on this subject at the World Congress of Biochemistry which took place in Moscow in 1972.

Current Physiological Understanding

1. CO_2 is, through the conversion into carbonic acid, the most important buffer system in the body's regulation of its acid-base balance (acid-alkali balance). A low level of CO_2 may lead to alkalosis. If the level of CO_2 lowers to below 3% shifting the pH to 8 then the whole organism dies.
2. A low level of CO_2 causes a displacement of the oxyhemoglobin dissociation curve, thereby not allowing correct oxygenation of the tissues and vital organs. (Bohr effect).

3. Poor oxygenation leads to hypoxia and a whole gamut of medical disorders.
4. CO_2 is a smooth muscle vessel dilator. Therefore a shortfall of CO_2 causes spasming of brain tissue, bronchus tissue etc.
5. Hyperventilation causes a progressive loss of CO_2. The higher the breathing, the lower the CO_2 level.
6. CO_2 is the catalyst to the body's metabolic processes, playing a vital role in biosynthesis of amino acids and their amides, Lipids, Carbohydrates, etc. This is explained in more detail in "The Biochemical Basis of K.P. Buteyko's Theory of the Disease of Deep Respiration".

Through an understanding of current physiology we should begin to see the links between CO_2 and oxygenation of the body, CO_2 and disease. It is clear that a deepening of the breathing does not mean an increase in oxygen uptake. On the contrary it means a decrease in oxygenation, which leads to hypoxia, imbalance in the acid-alkali balance, and cell spasming.

The fifth point of physiological understanding explains the destructively poisonous influence that hyperventilation has on the organism. It shows us clearly (in conjunction with the other points) that over-breathing leads to imbalance in the body and general deterioration of health.

The Dangers Of Hyperventilation

The term "hyperventilation" should be clearly defined. It is not reserved only to the most extreme and visible cases. Hyperventilation simply means "an increase in the function of the lungs above the normal recommended amount." The significance of Buteyko's discoveries hinge on the diagnosis of what Buteyko termed "hidden hyperventilation", that is long term over-breathing that is not clearly visible in the patient.

If a patient hyperventilating 30 Lt/min. can receive disastrous physical repercussions in the very short term, then it should be understood that over-breathing 5-10 Lt/min will have equally dire consequences over the long term. The average asthmatic over-breathes between 3 to 5 times the recommended amount, sometimes more.

The detrimental influence of the deep breathing on the organism is a direct result of the creation of a CO_2 deficit. This has been proven by many experiments, starting with the work of the well-known physiologist, Dr D Henderson, in 1909. In his experiments, animals were mechanically induced to deep breath and died as a result.

Acid-Alkali Balance

Through its conversion into carbonic acid, CO_2 is the most vital player in the maintaining of the body's acid-base balance. Lowering CO_2 in the lungs by deep breathing shifts the body's pH towards alkalinity, which changes the rate of activity of all body ferments and vitamins. An alkaline system is more 'susceptible to virus' and allergies. The shift in the rate of metabolic regulator activity disturbs the normal flow of metabolic processes and leads to the death of the cell. As mentioned before, if the level of CO_2 is lowered below 3%, shifting pH to 8, the whole of the organism dies.

Hyperventilation, Disease and Modern Medicine

Symptoms of various combined disturbances in the organism of a deep-breathing person are exceptionally diverse. The traditional methods of disease analysis have resulted in the various symptoms of over-breathing: (bronchospasms, heart muscle spasms, increased or decreased arterial pressures, fainting spells with convulsions) being called separate illnesses: bronchial asthma, stenocardia, hypertension, allergies, etc. The latter named all lead to complications, sclerosis of the lungs and vessels, myocardial infarcts, and strokes.

The theory of the diseases of deep breathing has previously been presented in a lecture: "On Discovery of the Deep Breathing Being the Principal Reason for Allergies, Sclerosis, Psychosis, Tuberculosis, Pre-cancerous Conditions and Other Symptoms of Disease."

In that lecture Professor Buteyko mentioned that his discovery is not only represented in the method of treatment of the diseases, but in the exposure of their causes. Professor Buteyko believes that modern medicine has slipped to the levels of blind empiricism. This appears to have happened because attempts to find the causes of diseases such as asthma, stenocardia, hypertension, etc., have been fruitless, therefore an important principle of medicine is being trampled on. The very principle upon which the Buteyko philosophy is based: "Having not found the reason of the disease, the physician has no right to treat the patient. Only having discovered the reason for the disease, is it possible to guarantee the recovery."

Modern medicine, as it stands at the moment, has either stopped looking for the causes of asthma, stenocardia, hypertension, etc, or it has a false impression of their reasons. That is why these diseases continue to remain incurable. Through understanding "trigger factors" we can only hope to treat the problem symptomatically. Only through the understanding of the cause of the disease, can we hope to cure.

It has eventuated, through Professor Buteyko's research, that deep breathing is directly linked to at least 150 diseases. Buteyko has conducted an immense synthesis of diseases and has found that diseases such as asthma, hypertension, stenocardia, myocardial infarcts, strokes, haemorrhoids, eczema, amongst others, are all symptoms of the imbalance created by deep breathing. In cases where Buteyko's patients had these diseases, they have all been cured, as was proven in the Leningrad and Moscow approbations [see page 160]. The Buteyko theory cites that these diseases are the body's defence mechanisms against the excessive loss of CO_2 through over-ventilation.

The Nervous System

The lowering of CO_2 in the nerve cells heightens the threshold of their excitability, alerting all branches of the nervous system and rendering it extraordinarily sensitive to outside stimuli. This leads to irritability, sleeplessness, stress problems, unfounded anxiety fears, allergic reactions, etc. Concurrent with this, the breathing centre in the brain is further stimulated thereby causing a further loss of CO_2. In this way another vicious cycle had commenced.

The Causes Of Deep Breathing

Having touched directly on the physiological problems of hyper-ventilation, and the resulting "blowing off" of CO_2, an obvious question arises: What is the cause of deep breathing itself? What is hyperventilation a consequence of?

There are several factors known to induce deepening of the breath. The most important factor, in Buteyko's opinion, is the propaganda of the usefulness of deep breathing. The contemporary man starts to be taught to breathe deeply even before he is born, when his mother is sent for sessions of deep breathing exercises during her pregnancy. Often the newly born is encouraged to increase his breathing by having his little arms raised and lowered. And so it follows on, in kindergartens, schools, armies, sport, etc. deep-breathing is encouraged without any scientific basis.

There are other factors as well – overeating, especially of animal protein (fish, chicken, eggs, milk and, naturally, meat) sharply increases breathing. It should be noted that the animal products increase the breathing more than plant products; cooked food more than raw.

Another factor deepening the breath is a state of limited mobility, lack of physical work or activity, idleness. Physical activity encourages the release of CO_2 from the cells, increasing its levels in the body. The breath is deepened by hydrodynamics, by bed rest regimes, by pro-longed horizontal positions (especially lying on the back), prolonged sleep. Recommendations for longer periods of sleep and even sleep therapy have never cured anybody. Most attacks of epilepsy, asthma, myocardial infarction, strokes, paralysis etc. occur towards the end of sleep, around 5am.

Further factors deepening the breath are the various emotions either positive or negative, stress, heat, stuffy environments. And the other way around, calmness, temperance, cold temperatures, all assist the shallow breathing.

The Aim of the Buteyko Method

The aim of the Buteyko method is to correct the patient's breathing pattern, that is recondition the breathing pattern to internationally recommended physiological levels. Through this process the shortfall of CO_2 is also rectified. The Buteyko process is completely safe and drug free.

In contrast to the dangers of low CO_2, if the depth of breathing is decreased to below normal and the level of CO_2 in the organism is above normal by 0.5-1.0%, there are no negative symptoms manifested. On the contrary, those afflicted with the heavy consequences of deep breathing, e.g. bronchial asthma, stenocardia, hypertension, develop symptoms of super-endurance with higher than normal levels of CO_2. The Buteyko clinics have been regularly observing this for the second decade now. It is evident that decreasing of the depth of breathing does not result in any kind of undesirable occurrences.

What is the normal or correct amount of air we should be breathing? This varies from person to person although on average 3-4 litres per minute.

***For a more comprehensive analysis of the physiological role of CO_2, please read: "The Biochemical Basis of K.P. Buteyko's Theory of the Disease of Deep Respiration."

asthma in New Zealand 1981–1983: a case control study. Lancet 1989: 1: 917–22

Davie, H. Modern medicine. A doctor's dissent. 1977

Donnell, P. Exercise-induced asthma: the protective role of CO_2 during swimming. Lancet 1991: 337: 179–80

Douthwaite, A. H. The Treatment of Asthma. H. K. Lewis, 130

Downes, S. article from Airways, summarised in The Beta Agonist Debate: New Insights. The Asthma Welfarer 1995 (vi) Vol 29 No 1 page 3

Drinkwater, H. Fifty Years of Medical Progress (1873–1922). London

Folgering H. & Snik, A. Hyperventilation Syndrome and Muscle Fatigue. Journal of Psychosomatic Research, Vol. 32, 1988

Gayrard, P., Orehek, J., Grimaud, C., Charpin, J. Bronchoconstrictor effects of a deep inspiration in patients with asthma American Review of Respiratory Diseases 1975: 111: 433–39

Gould, Donald The Medical Mafia

Graham, T. Self-management of asthma through normalisation of breathing. The role of breathing therapy. Paper distributed to delegates at National Asthma Conference, Brisbane, Australia, October 1996. Available through Asthma Foundation of Queensland

Haldane, J. S. The absorption and dissociation of CO_2 by human blood. 1905

—— The regulation of the lung-ventilation. Journal of Physiology V:32, 1905

—— Organism and environment as illustrated by the physiology of breathing. 1917.

Haldane, J. S. & Priestley, J. Respiration. 1935

Hall, Percy Asthma and its Treatments. Heinemann, 1930.

Hand, W. Magical Medicine. 1980 (first published 1907)

Herxheimer, Herbert G. J. The Management of Bronchial Asthma. Butterworth, 1952

Hibbert, G., Pilsbury, D. Demonstration and treatment of hyperventilation causing asthma. British Journal of Psychiatry 1988: 53: 687–89

Hopkins, A. Epilepsy. 1995

Hormbrey, J., et al CO_2 response and patterns of breathing in patients with symptomatic hyperventilation compared to asthmatic and normal subects. European Respiratory Journal 1988: 1: 846–52

Illich, Ivan Limits to Medicine

—— Medical Nemesis: The Exploitation of Health. 1976

Innocenti, Dr. 'Chronic Hyperventilation' in Text Book for Physiotherapists. London, 1986

Jain, S., Talukdar, B. Evaluation of Yoga Therapy Programme for Patients of Bronchial Asthma

The Results of the Approbation of the BBL Method in the Department of Children's Diseases in the First Moscow Medical Institute of E.M. Sechenov

by K.P. Buteyko & V.A.Genina

The BBL method was tested and approved by the medical institute of E. N. Sechenov between 27.2.81 and 21.5.81.

The method is based on a conscious decrease in deep breathing, and specifically designed for patients suffering from bronchial asthma. It is based on the fact that clinical results show improvement proportional to the decrease in lung ventilation.

Clinical characterisations of patients with bronchial asthma:
The experiment was based on patients suffering from regular asthma attacks (once a day or more) during the previous month. Some of the patients had severe asthma leading to asphyxia. The purpose of the experiment was to demonstrate the relationship between the major symptoms of the disease (bronchospasm, cough, nasal blockage and so on) and hyperventilation. The patients were asked to undergo a three stage hyperventilation test (developed by Professor Buteyko in 1968).

1. The test was conducted in a sitting position. The patients were asked

to use the BBL method. Correctly followed instructions yielded the following results;

In 1-5 minutes there was a decrease or disappearance of the symptoms of asthma; the patients experienced relief from asphyxia, wheezing, cough or rhinitis.

2. The second stage involved a reverse process; the patients were asked to breathe deeply for 15-60 seconds until the first symptoms of an attack.

3. The patients were asked to repeat the BBL and thus prevent the onset of the attack independently.

If the patients did not understand the relationship between the hyperventilation and the disease, the test was repeated. The test was not conducted if the patients took a bronchodilator 1.5-2 hours prior to the test. 52 patients between the ages of 3 and 15 were treated according to the BBL method: 36 boys (69%) and 16 girls (31%). See Table I

Of the 52 children, 34 (65%) were hospitalised, 18 (35%) were outpatients. 24 (46%) had atopic bronchial asthma. 22 (42%) had mixed bronchial asthma, and 6 (12%) had bacterial allergy bronchial asthma. The majority of the patients (36) had been suffering from this condition for up to 5 years, 12 for between 6-10 years and 4 from 11-15 years. The patients were divided into 3 categories: mild, severe and very severe (see Table V).

Table I – Age and sex distribution of patients

Group	Number	Sex	Age		
		M (F)	3-5	6-10	11-15
Hospital	34	24 (10)	2	18	14
Ambulatory	18	12 (6)	5	12	1
Total	52	36 (16)	7	30	15

Table II – Patient distribution according to degree of asthma

Group	Number	Degree/duration of illness					
		Mild test	%	Severe test	%	Very severe test	%
Hospital	34	0	0	24	70.6	10	29.4
Ambulatory	18	1	5.5	13	72.2	4	22.0
Total	52	1	1.9	37	71.1	14	26.9

According to patients' histories, 41 cases (79%) had had pneumonia 1-7 times. 4 (8%) were taking corticosteroids (prednisolone tablets) prior to the BBL treatment. 6 (11%) were physically handicapped, 9 (17%) were obese; all the children had bad posture, 11 (21%) had chest deformity. 33 of the children (64%) had allergic reactions to medications. 34 (65%) had allergic reactions to food and 25 (48%) had allergic reactions to dust. 27 (52%) suffered from rhinitis. 18 (35%) had Quinke's oedema. 47 (90%) had a predisposition to colds and flu. All had problems with breathing through the nose; 36 (69%) had chronic tonsillitis, 11 (21%) sinus problems. 23 (44%) had frequent headaches, all had palpitations and 13 (25%) had unstable body temperature.

Acute periods of their condition were accompanied by the following symptoms: 31 (59%) had sleeping problems, 16 (31%) had loss of appetite and 13 (25%) constipation. Of the 52 children, 47 (90%) were regular hospital patients and only 5 (10%) did not require hospitalisation.

Prior to the BBL treatment, all children had antibiotic treatment, all had to use bronchodilators, 37 (71.2%) were using [a cromoglycate drug] over prolonged periods, 15 (29%) were taking antihistamines. All these treatments were having little effect.

The course of the BBL treatment consisted of a daily training of 40 to 90 minutes exercise in the mornings under the supervision of the specialist; self training included 3 to 5 hours under the supervision of the instructor or the parents. The majority of the children mastered the method in 5 to 10 minutes: they were eager, disciplined and enthusiastic.

After 1 to 5 days of the BBL treatment, the patients were able to stop their asthma attacks, coughs, blocked noses and wheezing. The patients were encouraged to use the BBL method rather than their medication to overcome their attacks. Thirty-eight (73%) discontinued their medication as soon as they commenced the BBL method. Eight (15%) cut down their medication after 3 to 4 days. Steroid medications however were an exception. They had to be reduced gradually. The patients were allowed to take their medication in conjunction with the treatment only if they were unable to stop the attack after 10 to 15 minutes with the BBL method. For these cases, medication dosage was reduced by a factor of 2 to 3 and remained sufficient to stop the attack.

The results of the BBL method

Fifty-two children were observed for between 29 and 84 days. The results were based on the following criteria:

a) no improvement
b) some improvement (the degree of attacks is lessened together with a considerable reduction in medication).
c) considerable improvement (cessation of the heavy attacks. Slight traces of the disease or a total disappearance of the symptoms).

The results are listed in Table III

Table III – Results of the BBL method

Group	Considerable improvement	Some improvement	No change	Worse
Hospital	28 (82.4%)	6 (17.6%)	0	0
Ambulatory	15 (83.3%)	3 (16.6%)	0	0
Total	43 (82.7%)	9 (17.3%)	0	0

Forty-three (83%) of the patients showed considerable improvement and nine (17%) showed some improvement. There were no cases showing no improvement. The average period of hospitalisation was 16 days. All the patients with bronchial asthma (52) improved in the first four days. They could breathe freely through the nose and their coughs and wheezing disappeared. Fifteen experienced 'sanogenes' (self-cleansing) reactions, manifesting themselves through nervous excitement, chills, raised temperatures (up to 39°C), headaches, muscular pains, intestinal pains, chest pains, weakness and hypersecretion of mucus. Some experienced appetite loss, nausea, vomiting, thrist, excessive salivation (smelling of their medication) and increased urination and defecation. These reactions lasted from a few hours to two days and happened two to three times. The time in the condition of the patient was relative to the length of the controlled pause.

The clinical observations of the dynamics and the functions of the bronchi were researched simultaneously (using Tiffno tests and Rait scale). All the patients showed the following results during the first fourteen days of the BBL treatment.

As the control pause increased from 10 to 40 seconds, so did the concentrations of immunoglobulins A, M, G and E. Forced expiration volume (Rait's measuring scale) was raised from 36.7 to 173.2 (see Table IV). The acid-alkali balance of the blood normalised (it became less basic), the pCO_2 of the arterial blood increased from 24.6 to 36.3 mmHg. Control pause increased from 3.9 +/- 0.3 seconds to 31.4 +/- 4.7 seconds (see Table V).

Table IV – Change in lung capacity with the BBL treatment

State of illness	Number	Start point	40 mins	Time in days		
				7	14	30
Severe	14	37 (+/-8)	82 (+/-11)	117 (+/-15)	159 (+/-16)	—
Average	26	76 (+/-8)	121 (+/-8)	161 (+/-18)	173 (+/-10)	139 (+/-9)

Table V – Change in control pause with the BBL treatment

State of illnes	Number	Start point	40 mins	Time in days		
				7	14	30
Severe	14	2.9 (+/-.3)	12.4 (+/-1.4)	28.0 (+/-4.9)	24.5 (+/-4.5)	31.4 (+/-4.7)
Average	26	5.4 (+/-.7)	12.5 (+/-1.8)	24.0 (+/-3.9)	28.3 (+/-6.4)	31.4 (+/-4.7)

Patients with severe cases of asthma increased their lung capacities by 27%; the allergic resistance increased by 33% (see Table VI).

Table VI – Change in allergic resistance (AR), expiration speed (ES) and lung capacity (LC) with the BBL treatment

State of illness	Number	Time					
		Start			14 days		
		LC	AR	ES	LC	AR	ES
Severe	8	39.2	29.4	22.1	66.2	62.0	72.3
Average	15	55.3	48.0	51.0	80.0	78.3	85.3

Conclusion
1. The BBL method as suggested by Professor Buteyko helps to decrease the number and severity of attacks as well as the dosage of medication.
2. As a result of this therapy, the indicators of acid-alkali balance and lung ventilation improved.
3. The method may be taught to children from 3 years of age up, either in hospital or as outpatients.
4. This method is endured by children of any age over 3.
5. This method is most effective in acute periods of bronchial asthma in very ill patients.

A Summary of the Australian Buteyko Asthma Trial

A semi-blinded, randomized study trial comparing the effects of Buteyko breathing technique with a placebo breathing technique was funded by the Australian Association of Asthma Foundations.

It was conducted at the Mater Hospital in Brisbane, and was designed and monitored by some of Australia's foremost medical asthma specialists.

Severe asthma sufferers were randomly allocated into either the Buteyko group, or the Placebo group. This was done in such a way as to result in statistically equal groups in terms of asthma severity and drug usage.

The Buteyko group (19 people) was taught Buteyko, the placebo group (20 people) was given general asthma education, relaxation exercises, and was taught non-hyperventilation breathing exercises (abdominal breathing).

Patients kept diary cards at home scoring symptoms (3 = maximal symptoms, 0 = no symptoms), PEF, and medication usage.

Please note that all measurements are statistically significant unless otherwise stated.

Results at 6 Weeks

Beta Agonist Use
Buteyko Group decreased average agonist use by 90.1%. (From 1235ug to 134ug)
Placebo group decreased average agonist use by 5%. (From 1029ug to 978ug)

Inhaled steroid use
Buteyko Group average inhaled steroid use fell 12.5% from 1893ug to

1656ug.
Placebo Group average inhaled steroid use remained statistically the same at 1450ug to 1551ug.

Diary Card Symptom Scores
Buteyko Group decreased symptoms score by 50%.
Placebo Group decreased symptoms score by 15%.

Quality of Life Score – Impact of Asthma on Patient Lives
Dimensions measured were breathlessness, mood, impact on social activity, concern for the future.
Buteyko Group – 54% improvement, better in all dimensions.
Placebo Group – 24% worsening.

Summary at 6 Weeks
After 6 weeks Buteyko subjects used 90.% less beta-agonist (relief medication), felt substantially better in terms of breathlessness, mood, social activity and concerns about the future, had less symptoms, and as a group used less inhaled steroid.

Results at 3 Months
Beta-agonist use
Buteyko group had maintained decreased average use by 90%
Placebo group had increased average use by 9%

Inhaled Steroid Use
Buteyko group had decreased average use by 49%
Placebo group was statistically the same as before the trial

Diary card symptom scores
Buteyko group – 71% improvement
Placebo group – 14% improvement

Quality of Life Scores
Buteyko group had significant improvement that was still maintained at 8 months.

Follow up at 8 months
At 8 months the decrease in beta-agonist use in the Buteyko group had been maintained.

Discussion
This study showed that a group of severe asthmatics (averaging over 12 puffs of relief medication) were able to reduce their medication to an

average of just over 1 puff per day, simply by learning a different model for breathing. As well as reduced relief medication, the need for steroids was also significantly reduced. This is combined with massively reduced symptoms and greatly improved quality of life.

In this trial it was also attempted to monitor changes in CO_2 levels, changes in peak expiratory flow levels, and minute volume levels. Because of the relatively small sample size, the only statistically significant change among these measures of lung function was minute volume. Minute volume is an objective measure of the volume of air breathed at rest in one minute while stable. It is a consistent measure of the degree of hyperventilation of the patient. The Buteyko group average minute volume dropped from 14.0+6.5 litres, to 9.6+3.1 litres, which is a significant drop when compared to the placebo group. This change is exactly as predicted by Buteyko theory which states that a reduction in hyperventilation will result in reduction in symptoms of asthma and hayfever. (Correlation was found between the relative reduction in beta-agonist use in the Buteyko group and the relative reduction in Minute Volume, r=0.51, p=0.04).

This Trial Summary is taken from *The Buteyko Manual* by James Hooper, Buteyko Practitioner, Townsville, Australia, ph: 61 77 255160, fax: 61 77 255578; Email: hooper@ultra.net.au. *The Buteyko Manual* (ISBN 0 646 324195) is published by Instep International Press, 1996.

Glossary

Bronchial – to do with the lungs.

Bronchodilator – a drug which dilates the bronchial tubes, apparently facilitating breathing.

Bronchospasm – the involuntary contraction of the bronchial tubes which is part of the mechanism of an asthma attack.

Control pause – the length of time you can hold your breath after breathing out and not feel the need to breathe again. An ideal control pause is 60 seconds; a control pause of 15 or below denotes serious and chronic asthma.

Cromoglycate – a drug first marketed in the 1960s. it failed to achieve the 'miracle cure' status originally claimed for it, but is still commonly prescribed for children suffering from asthma.

Hyperventilation – overbreathing i.e. taking in more air than the internationally recognised physiological norm. It is a fundamental principle of Professor Buteyko's teaching that many diseases – and all asthma – are caused by hyperventilation.

Nebuliser – a method of administering bronchodilating drugs that is as much as 50 times more intense than the familiar 'puffer'.

Peak flow meter – a device used in conventional medicine to measure 'force-expiration' i.e. the amount of air you can blow out in one go.

Reliever medicine – one that relieves symptoms (such as bronchospasm in asthma) without attempting to prevent the disease.

Salbutamol – a commonly prescribed bronchodilator.

Steroid – a drug which is chemically similar to a natural hormone and which is commonly prescribed as an anti-inflammatory. Steroids are an important preventive treatment for asthma and can be given intravenously as an emergency treatment during an asthma attack.

References

Adam, James *Asthma and its Radical Treatment.* Kimpton, 1926

Adverse Drugs Reactions Bulletin, August 1994

Benson R. & Perlman F. *Clinical effects of epinephrine by inhalation.* Journal of Allergy 1948: 19: 129–140

Bhagat, R et al. *Salbutamol-induced increased airway responsiveness to allergen and reduced protein versus methacholine: dose response.* Journal of Allergy & Clinical Immunology 1996: Vol 1 Part 1

Blauw, G. & Westendrop, R. *Asthma Deaths in New Zealand: Whodunnit?* Lancet 1995: 345: 2–3

Bowler, S. D. , Green, A., Mitchell, C. A. *Buteyko breathing in asthma: a blind randomised controlled trial,* Mater Hospital, South Brisbane, Queensland. Medical Journal of Australia, Vol 169: 7/21 December 1998: 575–578

Brisco, Paula *Asthma: Questions You Have, Answers You Need.* Thorsons, 1997

British Medical Association *Fifty Years of Medicine.* London, 1950

Burney, P. G. J. *Strategy for Asthma.* BMJ 1991: 303, 571–3

Christian, H. A. & Mackenzie, J. (eds.) *The Oxford Medicine.*1932

Clarke, P. S. *Effect of disodium cromoglycate on exacerbations of asthma produced by hyperventilation.* BMJ 1971: 1: 317–19

—— *Asthma Hyperventilation and Emotion.* Australian Family Physician, 1980: Vol 9: October

Cochrane et al *A survey of asthma mortality in patients between ages 35 and 64 in the Greater London hospitals.* Thorax 1975: 30.

Coke, F. *Asthma.* Wright & Sons, 1923

Conybeare, J. J. *A Textbook of Medicine.* Livingstone, 1929

Corrigan, C. *Mechanism of glucocorticoid action in asthma; too little too late.* Clin. Exp. Allergy 1992: 22: 315–7

Crane, J., Pearce, N., Flatt, A. et al *Prescribed fenosterol and death from asthma in New Zealand 1981–1983: a case control study*. Lancet 1989: 1: 917–22

Davie, H. *Modern medicine. A doctor's dissent*. 1977

Donnell, P. *Exercise-induced asthma: the protective role of CO_2 during swimming*. Lancet 1991: 337: 179–80

Douthwaite, A. H. *The Treatment of Asthma*. H. K. Lewis, 130

Downes, S. article from *Airways,* summarised in *The Beta Agonist Debate: New Insights*. The Asthma Welfarer 1995 (vi) Vol 29 No 1 page 3

Drinkwater, H. *Fifty Years of Medical Progress (1873–1922)*. London

Folgering H. & Snik, A. *Hyperventilation Syndrome and Muscle Fatigue*. Journal of Psychosomatic Research, Vol. 32, 1988

Gayrard, P., Orehek, J., Grimaud, C., Charpin, J. *Bronchoconstrictor effects of a deep inspiration in patients with asthma* American Review of Respiratory Diseases 1975: 111: 433–39

Gould, Donald *The Medical Mafia*

Graham, T. *Self-management of asthma through normalisation of breathing. The role of breathing therapy*. Paper distributed to delegates at National Asthma Conference, Brisbane, Australia, October 1996. Available through Asthma Foundation of Queensland

Haldane, J. S. *The absorption and dissociation of CO_2 by human blood*. 1905

—— *The regulation of the lung-ventilation*. Journal of Physiology V:32, 1905

—— *Organism and environment as illustrated by the physiology of breathing*. 1917.

Haldane, J. S. & Priestley, J. *Respiration*. 1935

Hall, Percy *Asthma and its Treatments*. Heinemann, 1930.

Hand, W. *Magical Medicine*. 1980 (first published 1907)

Herxheimer, Herbert G. J. *The Management of Bronchial Asthma*. Butterworth, 1952

Hibbert, G., Pilsbury, D. *Demonstration and treatment of hyperventilation causing asthma*. British Journal of Psychiatry 1988: 53: 687–89

Hopkins, A. *Epilepsy*. 1995

Hormbrey, J., et al *CO_2 response and patterns of breathing in patients with symptomatic hyperventilation compared to asthmatic and normal subects*. European Respiratory Journal 1988: 1: 846–52

Illich, Ivan *Limits to Medicine*

—— *Medical Nemesis: The Exploitation of Health*. 1976

Innocenti, Dr. 'Chronic Hyperventilation' in *Text Book for Physiotherapists*. London, 1986

Jain, S., Talukdar, B. *Evaluation of Yoga Therapy Programme for Patients of Bronchial Asthma*

Lane, Donald J. *Asthma: The Facts*. 3rd edition, Oxford University Press 1996

Lask, Aaron *Asthma: Attitude and Milieu*. Tavistock Publications

Lasko, K. A. *The Great Billion Dollar Medical Swindle*

Lewis, K. H. & Howell, J. B. L. *Definition of the HVS*. Bulletin of European Physiopathology and Respiration, 1986: 22: 201

Mitchell, C., Bowler S. and Buteyko (Aust) P/L. *Agreement for Buteyko Trial,* November 1994

National Asthma Campaign, Melbourne: *Asthma Management Handbook*. 1993

Naughton M., Benard D., Rutherford R., Bradley T. *Effect of continuous positive airway pressure on central sleep apnoea and nocturnal PCO_2 in heart failure*. American Journal of Critical Care Medicine 1994: 1509, 1598–1604

New England Journal of Medicine, quoted in *The Asthma Welfarer* 1995, Vol 29: 1, 3

O'Donnell S. *The drug therapy of asthma – what are the outstanding questions?* Paper presented at National Asthma Conference, Brisbane, October 1996

Osler, W. *The Principles and Practice of Medicine*. Young J. Pentland, 1892

Pearce, N., Beasley R., Crane J. et al *End of the New Zealand asthma mortality epidemic*. Lancet 1995: 345: 41-44

Royal Society of Medicine *Nocturnal Asthma*. 1984

Salter, Henry Hyde *Asthma: Its Pathology and Treatment*. Churchill, 1860

Sears M. et al. *75 deaths in asthmatics prescribed home nebulisers*. British Medical Journal 1987: 294

Sears M., Taylor D., Print C. et al *Regular inhaled salbutamol may exacerbate bronchial inflammation in patients with mild asthma*. Thorax 1993: 48: 1060

Selroos O et al. *Effect of early vs late intervention with inhaled corticosteroids in asthma*. Chest 1988: 108: 1228–34

Serafini, U. *Can fatal asthma be prevented? – a personal view*. Clin. Exp. Allergy 1992, 22: 576–88

Serevent: Long-acting inhaler for asthma. Medical Sciences Bulletin, June 1994. Pharmaceutical Information Associates Ltd

Speizer et al. *Observations on recent increase in mortality from asthma*. BMJ 1968: 1

—— *Investigation into use of drugs preceding death from asthma*. BMJ 1986: 1

Tobin, M. J. et al *Breathing Patterns. Diseased Subjects*. Chest, 1963: 84: 287–94

Van den Elshout, F., van Herwaarden, J., Folgering, H. *Effects of hypercapnia and hypocapnia on respiratory resistance in normal and asthmatic subject.* 1991. Thorax 46: 28–32

West, B. *Respiratory Physiology.* 4th edition, Williams & Williams, 1990

Wilbur, R. L. *The March of Medicine.* Stanford, 1938

Woolcock, A. J. and Read, J. *Improvement in asthma not reflected in forced expiratory volume.* The Lancet 1965: 2: 1323.

Youngson, Dr Robert *Living with Asthma.* Sheldon Press, 1995

Index